YOGA VASISTHA,
AN INSTRUCTIONAL BOOK ON
HATHA YOGA
AND GUIDE TO
PHYSICAL WELL-BEING
THRU ANCIENT WISDOM OF
THE SCIENCE OF YOGA

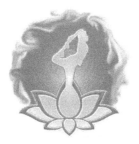

अथ योगानुशासनम् ॥१॥
atha yoga-anusăsanam

(now, the introduction to the
study and practice of yoga)

ISBN: 978-9491911002
2017, 1st edition

email
publish@white-mountains.eu
www.white-mountains.eu

Om Saha Năvavatu
Saha Nau Bhunaktu
Saha Vĭryam Karavăvahai
Tejasvi năvadhĭtamastu
Mă Vidviṣăvahai

Om
Śăntih
Śăntih
Śăntih

ᑌᕳ CONTENTS ᕰᑌ

Preface
About the author
Yoga Vasistha

Preface

THIS book is dedicated to that part of Yoga which deals with the development and attainment of a healthy physical constitution. The information gathered in this book is a passing on of old knowledge in an effort to make it accessible to people from all walks of life.

Within the framework of the Science of Yoga this knowledge and instructions is called 'Hatha Yoga' and lies at the root of Yoga and its Higher Teachings. This knowledge comes naturally to each of us as our Instinctual Birth right. Often, through external influences like modern ways of living or misguided teaching, this Instinct has been derailed, diluted or changed during the course of lives, creating confusion later on when it seems impossible to return to these Natural ways. This book hopes to achieve a refreshing of this knowledge in its readers, where applicable fill in gaps, a correcting of strayed habits and bring to light Yogi Knowledge that has been passed on through the ages. That this knowledge be cemented into your hearts, where it may form a solid base to be used in your everyday lives and act as an incentive to pursue further along the Path of Wisdom of the Ancient Yogis.

It is emphasized that any literature found concerning the Science of Yoga goes best accompanied with a discourse by a competent and skilled teacher in the subject matter. Guidance into the philosophical aspects of the Science of Yoga is important, and no physical exercise should be performed without prior first-hand instructions, at the risk of misinterpretation, doing more harm than good.

About the author

THE grace of universal wisdom is such that it cares not for background, upbringing, society, culture, caste, race, intellect, learning, achievements, religion, conviction, geographical location or any other definition that labels us thus. Universal Wisdom is available for each of us who cares to be receptive and willing to embrace the knowledge that comes forth if we but allow ourselves to be open. As unlikely as it may seem —the author of this book has come from an entirely different background you would expect from a Yogi— life's experiences have led him to the same understandings and uncovering of Universal Truths as all Yogis have through the ages. These, in turn, can be found in the ancient Wisdom of Yoga.

As a young boy, Ernest van der Linden was always more eager to venture out and experience life on his own terms, than follow the rules imposed by society in the West where he was born. That attitude soon brought him to many places around the world at an early age, eagerly adapting to local cultures and habits, learning languages and traits that would sustain his life at such a particular moment in time and space. This lifestyle forced a reconsideration of his approach to life numerous times, which at one point led Ernest to pursue a more traditional career.

Not hindered by doctrines his contemporaries had accumulated in elaborate and rigid studies and conventional jobs, Ernest found himself at the world-top of his trade within just a few years at a young age, an achievement that traditionally takes decades of hard work and study to accomplish—if ever. Only to find that what society proclaims to be the ultimate goal of such a career—such a life indeed, is to live life as in a mausoleum. For Ernest, the only way forward was to break away from all these societies' so sought after boons like fame, fortune, status etcetera.

Thereafter, finding no answers within all his life's experiences for a further course in life he realized to have stumbled upon a dead end, and had but one course of action left—to 'LET GO' of all the accumulated beliefs, convictions and doctrines that remained.

That final 'Letting Go' made room for Universal Truths to enter his consciousness. Ernest's pursuit to know more about that experience and the knowledge attained therein, inspired him to create this small book in hopes it may work as a stepping stone onto the path of Yoga for some, or as an inspiration to lead healthy lives for others. Ernest himself is treading a steady and firm pace on the path of the Ancient Yogis, finding no better roadmap to good health and unfoldment elsewhere than through the Science of Yoga.

By contrast to this work, there is one suggestion Ernest would like to make in terms of literature, and that is for you to pick up and read a copy of 'The Bhagavad Gita' (The Song Divine).

A special thanks is owed to Sunilkumar Ramachandran, native to South India, Kerala. Sunil has been practicing yoga since the 1980s' and started teaching since 1998 to thousands of students from all over the world. Because of his studies in yoga, its philosophy and the many spiritual aspects associated, his classes are not exercises. It is rejuvenation for the body, the mind, the spirit. Sunil is famous for his savăsana instruction and his gentle approach to correct postures. Sunil is teaching in his own center 'Yoga Vasishta' at Varkala Beach in Kerala, offering the exact sequence of ăsanas you will find in the daily yoga routine included at the end of this book.

Yoga Vasistha

YOGA VASISTHA' was a Hindu spiritual text written by a sage called Valmiki and is believed to answer all the questions that arise in the human mind, and can help one to attain Moksha (liberation from rebirth). The Yoga Vasistha recounts a discourse of sage Vasistha to Prince Rama when he is in a dejected state. Prince Rama returns from touring the country, and becomes utterly disillusioned after experiencing the apparent reality of the world. This worries his father, King Dasaratha, who expresses his concern to Sage Vasistha. Sage Vasistha consoles the king by telling him that Rama's dis-passion (vairagya) is a sign that the prince is now ready for spiritual enlightenment. He says that Rama has begun understanding profound spiritual truths, which is the cause of his confusion; he needs confirmation. Sage Vasistha asks the king to summon Rama. Then, in King Dasaratha's court, the sage begins his discourse to Rama. The answer to Rama's questions forms the scripture called 'Yoga Vasistha.' It is one of the longest texts in Sanskrit after the Mahabharata, and an important text of Yoga. It consists of about 32,000 shlokas (verses), including numerous short stories and anecdotes used to help illustrate its content.

The choice to make the name 'Vasistha' part of this books' title is not intended to imply that what the Yoga Vasistha contains is herein translated or covered. The inclusion was inspired by the Yogi Wisdom the old text holds and hence the name implies. The original work is written in the Sanskrit language, not accessible to many, and whilst this book imparts part of that knowledge in plain language, the reference to the ancient scripture seemed appropriate.

The Yogi Philosophy of Physical Well-Being

THIS book is dedicated to that part of the Science of Yoga that deals with our physical aspects: 'Hatha Yoga', or 'The Yogi Philosophy of Physical Well-Being.' Before diving into our subject matter, it will be good to have a brief introduction to the Philosophy of Yoga, and see how our subject matter fits into this great 'Science of Yoga.'

The Yogi Philosophy may be divided into several great branches. Among the best-known and leading divisions are Raja Yoga, Karma Yoga, Gnani Yoga and Bhakti Yoga. Each of these forms of Yoga being travelled by those who may prefer it—but all leading to the one end-unfoldment, development, and growth. The aim is to bring the unconscious and subconscious to conscious perception—in Union (Yoga).

The Great Branches of Yoga

RAJA YOGA' is devoted to the development of the latent powers in Man—the gaining of the control of the mental faculties by the Will—the attainment of the mastery of the lower self—the development of the mind to the end that the soul may be aided in its unfoldment. It teaches the care and control of the body, as taught in 'Hatha Yoga,' believing that the body should become an efficient instrument, and under good control, before the best results may be attained along mental and psychic lines.

KARMA YOGA' is the 'Yoga' of Work. It is the path followed by those who delight in their work, who take a keen interest in 'doing things' with head or hand—those who believe in work 'for work's sake.' 'Karma' is the Sanskrit word applied to the 'Law of Spiritual Cause and Effect.' Karma Yoga teaches how one may go through life working—and taking an interest in action—without being influenced by selfish consideration, which might create a fresh chain of cause and effect that would bind him to objects and things, and thus hold back his spiritual progress. It teaches 'work for work's sake' rather than from a desire for results.

GNANI YOGA' is the 'Yoga of Wisdom.' It is followed by those of a scientific, intellectual type, who are desirous of reasoning out, proving, experimenting, and classifying the occult knowledge. It is the path of the scholar. Its follower is strongly attracted toward metaphysics. Examples of the idea of 'Gnani Yogi'—apparently widely differing examples—are to be seen in the great philosophers of ancient and modern times, and in the other extreme, those who have a strong tendency toward metaphysical teachings.

BHAKTI YOGA' is really what we might call the 'religious' form of Yoga, teaching the love and worship of God, according to how he appears to us through the colored glasses of our own particular creed. Some treat what is known as 'Bhakti Yoga ' as if it were a separate path, but we prefer thinking of it as being an incident of each of the other three paths.

It must not be supposed that the student must ally himself to only a single one of these paths. In fact, very few do. The majority prefers to gain a rounded knowledge, and acquaint themselves with the principles of the several branches, learning something of each, giving preference of course to those branches that appeal to them more strongly, this attraction being the indication of _need_, or requirement, and, therefore, being the hand pointing out the path.

What is 'Hatha Yoga?'

HATHA YOGA' is that branch of the Yogi Philosophy that deals with the physical body—its care—it's well-being—its health—its strength— and all that tends to keep it in its natural and normal state of health. It teaches a natural mode of living and voices the cry that has been taken up by many;

"Let Us Get Back To Nature."

The Yogi clings close to nature and her ways, and will not be dazzled and fooled by the mad rush toward externals, which has caused the modern civilized races to forget that such a thing as nature exists. Fashions and social ambitions do not reach the Yogi's consciousness—he smiles at these things, and regards them as he does the pretences of childish games—he has not been lured from nature's arms, but continues to cuddle close up to the bosom of his good mother who has always given him nourishment, warmth and protection.

Hatha Yoga is first; nature, second; nature, and last; NATURE.

When confronted with a choice of methods, plans, theories, etcetera, along health lines with which the world is being flooded, apply to them the touchstone: 'Which is the natural way,' and always choose that which seems to conform the nearest to nature—and if they do not square with nature, discard them—it is a safe rule. Nature knows what it is about—she is your friend and not your enemy.

Hatha Yoga preaches a sane, natural, normal manner of living and life which, if followed, will benefit any one. It keeps close to nature and advocates a return to natural methods in preference to those that have grown up around us in our artificial habits of living. The underlying principle of Hatha Yoga—belief in the Intelligence behind all Life—to have trust in the great Life Principle to carry on its work properly; the belief that if we will but rely on that great principle, and will allow it to work in and through us, all will be well with our bodies.

In answer to the question with which this chapter is headed: "What is Hatha Yoga?", we say to you: Read this book to the end, and you will understand some little about what it really is—to find out all it is put into practice the precepts of this book, and you will get a good fair start on the road to that knowledge you seek.

The Physical Body

THE Yogis believe that real Man is not his body. They know that the immortal 'I' of which each human being is conscious to a greater or lesser degree, is not the body, which it merely occupies and uses. They know that the body is but as a suit of clothes which the Spirit puts on and off from time to time. They know the body for what it is, and are not deceived into the belief that it is the real Man. But while knowing these things, they also know that the body is the instrument in which, and by which the Spirit manifests and works. They know that the fleshly covering is necessary for Man's manifestation and growth in this particular stage of his development. They know that the body is the Temple of the Spirit. And they, consequently, believe that the care and development of the body is as worthy a task as is the development of some of the higher parts of Man, for with an unhealthy and imperfectly developed physical body, the mind cannot function properly, nor can the instrument be used to the best advantage by its master, the Spirit.

For these reasons, the Yogi pays such great attention and care to the physical side of his nature. The highly trained body must, first of all be a strong healthy body. The Yogi throws Mind into the task, and develops not only the muscle but every organ, cell, and part of his body as well. Not only does he do this, but he obtains control over every part of his body, and acquires mastery over the involuntary part of his organism as well as over the voluntary. He insists that the body be brought under the perfect control of the mind—that the instrument be finely turned so to be responsive to the touch of the master.

The Divine Architect

THE Yogi Philosophy teaches that each individual is given a physical machine adapted to his needs, and also supplied with the means of keeping it in order, and of repairing it if his negligence allows it to become inefficient. The Yogis recognize the human body as the handiwork of a great Intelligence. They regard its organism as a working machine, the conception and operation of which indicates the greatest wisdom and care. They know that the body IS because of a great Intelligence, and they know that the same Intelligence is still operating through the physical body, and that as the individual falls in with the working of the Divine Law, so will he continue in health and strength. They also know that when Man runs contrary to that law, disharmony and disease result. They believe it is ridiculous to suppose that this great Intelligence caused the beautiful human body to exist, and then ran away and left it to its fate, for they know that the Intelligence still presides over each and every function of the body, and may be safely trusted and not feared.

That Intelligence, the manifestation of which we call 'Nature' or 'The Life Principle,' and similar names, is constantly on the alert to repair damage, heal wounds, knit together broken bones; to throw off harmful materials which have accumulated in the system; and in thousands of ways to keep the machine in good running order. Much that we call disease is really a beneficent action of Nature designed to get rid of poisonous substances which we have allowed to enter and remain in our system.

It is well worth the time of anyone to study something of the wonderful mechanism and workings of the human body. One gets from this study a most convincing realization of the reality of that great Intelligence in nature—he sees the great Life Principle in operation—he sees that it is not blind chance, or haphazard happening, but that it is the work of a mighty INTELLIGENCE.

Then he learns to trust that Intelligence, and to know that that which brought him into physical being will carry him through life—that the power which took charge of him then, has charge of him now, and will have charge of him always.

As we open ourselves to the inflow of the great Life Principle, so will we be benefited. If we fear it, or trust it not, we shut the door upon it and must necessarily suffer.

The Vital Force

MANY people make the mistake of considering Disease as an entity—a real thing—an opponent of Health. This is incorrect. Health is the natural state of Man, and disease is simply the absence of Health. If one can comply with the laws of Nature, he cannot be sick. When some law is violated, abnormal conditions result, and certain symptoms manifest themselves, and to which symptoms we give the name of some disease. That which we call disease is simply the result of Nature's attempt to throw off, or dislodge, the abnormal condition, in order to resume normal action.

Nature is not fickle or unreliable. Life manifests itself within the body in pursuance to well established laws, and pursues its way, slowly, rising until it reaches its zenith, then gradually going down the decline until the time comes for the body to be thrown off like an old, well-used garment, when the soul steps out on its mission of further development. Nature never intended that a man should part with his body until a ripe old age was attained, and the Yogis know that if Nature's laws were observed from childhood, the death of a young or middle-aged person from disease would be as rare as is death from accident.

There is within every physical body, a certain vital force which is constantly doing the best it can for us, notwithstanding the reckless way in which we violate the cardinal principles of right living. Much of that which we call disease is but a defensive action of this vital force—a remedial effect. It is not a downward action but an upward action on the part of the living organism. The action is abnormal, because the conditions are abnormal, and the whole recuperative effort of the Vital Force is exerted toward the restoration of normal conditions.

The first great principle of the Vital Force is self-preservation. This principle is ever in evidence, wherever life exists. Under its action the male and female are attracted—the embryo and infant are provided with nourishment—the mother is caused to bear heroically the pains of maternity—the parents are impelled to shelter and protect their offspring under the most adverse circumstances—Why? Because all this means the instinct of race-preservation.

But the instinct of preservation of individual life is equally strong. "All that a man hath will he give for his life," said the writer, and while it is not strictly true of the developed man, it is sufficiently true to use for illustrating the principle of self-preservation. And this instinct is not of the Intellect, but is found down among the foundation stones of being. It is an instinct which often overrules Intellect. It makes a man's legs 'run away with him' when he had firmly resolved to stand in a dangerous position— it causes a shipwrecked man to violate some of the principles of civilization, causing him to kill and eat his comrade and drink his blood— it has made wild beasts of men and under many and varying conditions it asserts supremacy. It is working always for life—more life—for health—

more health. And it often makes us sick in order to make us healthier—brings on a disease in order to get rid of some foul matter which our carelessness and folly has allowed to intrude in the system.

This principle of self-preservation on the part of the Vital Force moves us along in the direction of health, as surely as does the influence within the magnetic needle make it point due north. We may turn aside, not heeding the impulse, but the urge is always there. The same instinct is within us, which, in the seed, causes it to put forth its little shoot, often moving weights a thousand times heavier than itself, in its effort to get to the sunlight. The same impulse causes the sapling to shoot upward from the ground. The same principle causes roots to spread downward and outward. In each case, although the direction is different, each move is in the right direction. If we are wounded, the Vital Force begins to heal the wound, doing the work with wonderfully good judgement and precision. If we break a bone, all that we or the surgeon may do, is to place the bones into juxtaposition and keep them there, while the great Vital Force knits the fractured parts together. If we fall, or our muscles or ligaments are torn, all that we can do is to observe certain things in the way of attention, and the Vital Force starts in to do its work, and drawing on the system for the necessary materials, repairs the damage.

All physicians know, and their schools teach, that if a man is in good physical condition, his Vital Force will cause him to recover from almost any condition excepting when the vital organs are destroyed. When the physical system has been allowed to run down, recovery is much more difficult, if, indeed, not impossible, as the efficiency of the Vital Force is impaired and is compelled to work under unfavorable conditions. But rest assured that it is doing the best it can for you, always, under the existing conditions. If Vital Force cannot do for you all that it aims to do, it will not give up the attempt as hopeless, but will accommodate itself to circumstances and make the best of it. Give it a free hand and it will keep you in perfect health—restrict it by irrational and unnatural methods of living, and it will still try to pull you through, and will serve you until the end, to the best of its ability, in spite of your ingratitude and stupidity. It will fight for you to the finish.

We are living in a civilization which has forced a more or less unnatural mode of life upon us, and the Vital Force finds it hard to do as well for us as it would like. We do not eat naturally; drink naturally; sleep naturally; breathe naturally; or dress naturally. We "have done those things which we ought not to have done, and we have left undone those things which we ought to have done, and there is no Health within us" or, we might add, as little health as we can help.

We have dwelt upon the matter of the friendliness of the Vital Force, for the reason that it is a matter usually overlooked by those who have not made a study of it. It forms a part of the Yogi Philosophy of Hatha Yoga, and the Yogis take it largely into consideration in their lives. They know that they have a good friend and a strong ally in the Vital Force, and they allow it to flow freely through them, and try to interfere as little as possible with its operations. They know that the Vital Force is ever awake to their well-being and health, and they keep the greatest confidence in it.

Much of the success of Hatha Yoga consists of methods best calculated to allow the Vital Force to work freely and without hindrance, and its methods and exercises are largely devoted to that end. To clear the track of obstructions, and to give the chariot of the Vital Force the right of way on a smooth clear road, is the aim of the Hatha Yogi. Follow his precepts and it will be well with your body.

The Cell–Lives of The Body

HATHA Yoga teaches that the physical body is built up of cells, each cell containing within it a miniature 'life' which controls its action. These 'lives' are really bits of intelligent mind of a certain degree of development, which enable the cells to do their work properly. These bits of intelligence are, of course, subordinate to the control of the central mind of man, and readily obey orders given from headquarters, consciously or unconsciously. These cell intelligences manifest a perfect adaption for their particular work. The selective action of the cells, extracting from the blood the nourishment required, and rejecting that which is not needed is an instance of this intelligence. The process of digestion, assimilation, etcetera, shows the intelligence of the cells, either separately or collectively, in groups. The healing of wounds, the rush of the cells to the points where they are most needed, and hundreds of other examples known to the investigators, all mean to the Yogi student examples of the 'life' within each atom. Each atom is to the Yogi a living thing, leading its own independent life. These atoms combine into groups for some end, and the groups manifest a group-intelligence, so long as it remains a group; these groups again combining in turn, and forming bodies of a more complex nature, which serve as vehicles for higher forms of consciousness.

When death comes to the physical body, the cells separate and scatter and that which we call decay sets in. The force which has held the cells together is withdrawn, and they become free to go their own way and to form new combinations. Some go into the body of the plants in the vicinity, and eventually find themselves in the body of an animal; others remain in the organism of the plant; others remain in the ground for a time, but the life of the atom means incessant and constant change. As a leading writer has said:

"Death is but an aspect of life, and the destruction of one material form is but a prelude to the building up of another."

The cells of the body have three principles: (1) Matter, which they obtain from the food; (2) Prana, or vital force, which enables them to manifest action, and which is obtained from the food we eat; the water we drink and the air we breathe; (3) Intelligence, or 'mind-stuff,' which is obtained from the Universal Mind.

In the lower animals Nature allows the Instinctive Mind a fuller scope and a larger field, and as life ascends in the scale, developing the reasoning faculties, the Instinctive Mind seems to narrow its field. For instance, crabs and members of the spider family are able to grow new feeders, legs, claws, etc. Snails are able to grow even parts of the head, including eyes which have been destroyed; some fishes are able to re-grow tails. Salamanders and lizards are able to grow new tails, including bones, muscle and parts of the spinal column. The very lowest forms of animal life have practically an unlimited power of restoring lost parts and can practically make themselves entirely over, provided there is left the smallest part of them to build upon. The higher forms of animals have lost much of this recuperative power and man has lost more than any of them owing to his mode of living. Some of the more advanced of the Hatha Yogis, however, have performed some wonderful results along these lines, and any one, with patient practice, may obtain such control of the Instinctive Mind and the cells under its control that he may obtain wonderful recuperative results in the direction of renewing diseased parts and weakened portions of the body.

The cell-mind is supplied from the Universal Mind—the great storehouse of 'mind-stuff'—and is kept in touch and directed by the mind of the cell-centres, which are in turn controlled by higher centres, until the central Instinctive Mind is reached. But the cell-mind is not able to express itself without both of two other principles—matter and prana. It needs the fresh material supplied by the well-digested food, in order to make for itself a medium of expression. It also needs a supply of Prana, or Vital Force, in order to move and have action. The triune principle of Life—mind, matter and force—is necessary in the cell as in the man. Mind needs force or energy (prana) in order to manifest itself in action through matter.

Control of the Involuntary System

THE higher Yogis have a wonderful control over the involuntary system and can act directly upon nearly every cell in their body. The trained will is able to act directly upon cells and groups by a simple process of direct concentration, but this plan requires much training on the part of the student. There are other plans whereby the will is called into operation by repeating certain words in order to focus the Will. Auto-suggestions and affirmations of the Western world act in this way. The words focus the attention and Will upon the centre of the trouble and gradually order is restored among the striking cells, a supply of prana also being projected to the seat of the trouble, thus giving the cells additional energy. At the same time the circulation to the affected region is increased, thereby giving the cells more nourishment and building material.

One of the simplest plans of reaching the seat of trouble and giving a vigorous order to the cells is the one taught by the Hatha Yogis to their students, to be used by them until they are able to use the concentrated Will without any aids. The plan is simply to 'talk up' to the rebellious organ or part, giving it orders just as one would a group of school boys or a squad of recruits in the army. Give the order positively and firmly, telling the organ just what you wish it to perform, repeating the command sharply several times. A tapping or mild slapping of the part, or the part of the body over the affected part, will act to attract the attention of the cell-group just as does the tapping of a man on the shoulder cause him to stop, turn around and listen to what you have to say. Now, please do not suppose that we are trying to tell you that the cells have ears and understand the words of the particular language you may be using. What really happens is that the sharply spoken words help you to form the mental image expressed by the words, and this meaning goes right to the spot, over the channels of the sympathetic nervous system operated by the Instinctive Mind, and is readily understood by the cell-groups and even by the individual cells. As has already been said, an additional supply of prana and the increased supply of blood also go to the affected region, being directed there by the concentrated attention of the person sending the command. The commands of a healer may be given in the same way, the Instinctive Mind of the patient taking up the command and forwarding it to the scene of the cell rebellion. This may seem almost childish to many students, but there are good scientific reasons behind it, and the Yogis consider it the simplest plan whereby mental commands may reach the cells. So do not discard it as worthless until you have tried it awhile. It has stood the test of centuries, and nothing better has been found to do the work.

You will be surprised at the measure of control which you may gain over your body by following the above method and variations of the same.

Prana

PRANA is interwoven with the entire Hatha Yoga Philosophy, and must be seriously considered by its students. This being the case, we must consider the question,

"What is prana?"

Occultists in all ages and lands have always taught, usually secretly to a few followers, that there was to be found in the air, in water, in the food, in the sunlight, everywhere, a substance or principle from which all activity, energy, power and vitality was derived. They differed in their term and names for this force, as well as in the details of their theories, but the main principle is to be found in all occult teachings and philosophies, and has for centuries past been found among the teachings and practices of the Yogis. We have preferred to designate this vital principle by the name by which it is known among the Hindu teachers and students, gurus and chelas—and have used for this purpose the Sanskrit word 'Prana,' meaning 'Absolute Energy.'

Occult authorities teach that 'prana' is the universal principle of energy or force, and that all energy or force is derived from that principle, or, rather, is a particular form of manifestation of that principle. We may consider it as the active principle of life—Vital Force, if you please. It is found in all forms of life, -from the most elementary form of plant life to the highest form of animal life. Prana is all pervading. It is found in all things having life and as the occult philosophy teaches that life is in all things—in every atom—the apparent lifelessness of some things being only a lesser degree of manifestation, we may understand their teachings that prana is everywhere, in everything.

This great principle is in all forms of matter, and yet it is not matter. It is in the air, but it is not the air, nor one of its chemical constituents. It is in the food we eat, and yet it is not the same as the nourishing substances in the food. It is in the water we drink, and yet it is not one or more of the chemical substances which combining make water. It is in the sunlight, but yet it is not the heat or the light rays. It is the 'energy' in all these things— the things acting merely as a carrier.

And man is able to extract it from the air, food, water, sunlight and turn it to good account in his own organism. We are constantly inhaling the air charged with prana, and are constantly extracting the latter from the air and appropriating it to our uses. Prana is found in its freest state in the atmospheric air, which when fresh is fairly charged with it, and we draw it to us more easily from the air than from any other source. In ordinary breathing we absorb and extract a normal supply of prana, but by controlled and regulated breathing (generally known as Yogi breathing) we are enabled to extract a greater supply, which is stored away in the brain and nerve centers, to be used when necessary.

We may store away prana, just as the storage battery stores away electricity. The many powers attributed to advanced occultists are due largely to their knowledge of this fact and their intelligent use of this stored-up energy. The Yogis know that by certain forms of breathing they establish certain relations with the supply of prana and may draw on the same for what they require. Not only do they strengthen all parts of their body in this way, but the brain itself may receive increased energy from the same source, and latent faculties be developed and psychic powers attained. One who has mastered the science of storing away prana, either consciously or unconsciously, often radiates vitality, and strength which is felt by those coming in contact with him, and such a person may impart this strength to others, and give them increased vitality and health. What is called 'magnetic healing' is performed in this way, although many practitioners are not aware of the source of their power.

Western scientific theories regarding the breath confine themselves to the effects of the absorption of oxygen, and its use through the circulatory system, while the Yogi theory also takes into consideration the absorption of prana, and its manifestation through the channels of the Nervous System. Every thought, every act, every effort of the will, every motion of a muscle, uses up a certain amount of what is known to Western science as 'nerve force,' which the Yogi knows to be a manifestation of prana. In character and rapidity it resembles the electric current. Without this 'nerve force' the heart cannot beat; the blood cannot circulate; the lungs cannot breathe; the various organs cannot function; in fact, the machinery of the body comes to a stop without it. When it is remembered that the greater portion of prana acquired by man comes to him from the air inhaled, the importance of proper breathing is readily understood and the Yogi Science of Breath of which we will speak later assumes an even greater importance.

The Yogi teachings go further than does Western science in one important feature of the Nervous System. We hint at what Western science terms the 'Solar Plexus,' and which it considers as merely one of a series of certain matted nets of sympathetic nerves with their ganglia found in various parts of the body. Yogi Science teaches that this Solar Plexus is really a most important part of the Nervous System, and that it is a form of brain, playing one of the principal parts in the human economy. We will not go into the Yogi theory regarding the Solar Plexus, further than to say that they know it as the great central storehouse of prana. The name 'Solar' is well bestowed on this 'brain,' as it radiates strength and energy to all parts of the body, even the upper brains depending largely upon it as a storehouse of prana.

Nourishment

THE human body is constantly undergoing change. Atoms of bone, tissue, flesh, muscle, fat and fluids are constantly being worn out and removed from the system, and new atoms are constantly being manufactured in the wonderful laboratory of the body, and then sent to take the place of the worn out and discarded material.

This great work of discarding worn out material and the substitution of new material goes on constantly, day and night. We are not conscious of this mighty work, as it belongs to that great subconscious part of Man's nature—it is a part of the work of the Instinctive Mind.

The whole of the body, and all its parts, depend for health, strength and vigour upon this constant renewal of material. If this renewal were stopped disintegration and death would ensue. The replacing of the worn out and discarded material is an imperative necessity of our organism, and, therefore, is the first thing to be considered when we think of the Healthy Man. The keynote of this subject of replacing this discarded material in the Hatha Yoga Philosophy is 'NOURISHMENT.'

The Yogis, at least those who are well-grounded in Hatha Yoga, regard Nourishment as his first duty towards his body, and he is always careful to keep that body properly nourished, and to see that the supply of new, fresh material is always at least equal to the worn out and discarded matter. A maxim of Hatha Yoga is:

'It is not what a man eats, but the amount that he assimilates, that nourishes him.'

There is a world of wisdom in this old maxim, and it contains that which writers upon health subjects have taken volumes to express.

To the Yogi, food does not mean something to tickle the abnormal palate. The Yogi has cultivated and encouraged his natural and normal taste so that his hunger imparts to the plainest food a relish sought after, but not obtained, by those who hunt after rich and expensive triumphs of the chef. While eating for Nourishment as his main object, he manages to make his food yield him a pleasure unknown to his brother who scorns the simple fare.

Hunger vs. Appetite

HUNGER and appetite are two entirely different attributes of the human body. Hunger is the normal demand for food—Appetite the abnormal craving. Hunger is like the rosy hue upon the cheek of the healthy child—Appetite is like the rouged face of the woman of fashion. And yet most people use the terms as if their meaning were identical.

To one who has set himself free from the thrall of appetite, the respective sensations of Hunger and Appetite are quite different, and the mind of such a person grasps the precise meaning of each term without difficulty. But to the ordinary 'civilized' man 'Hunger' means the source of appetite and 'Appetite' the result of hunger. Both words are misused.

Let us take Thirst. All of us know the sensation of a good, natural thirst, which calls for a draught of cool water. It is felt in the mouth and throat, and can be satisfied only with that which Nature intended for it— cool water. Now, this natural Thirst is akin to natural Hunger.

We hear people say that they are 'so thirsty' for a glass of soda-water; or others say that they are 'thirsty' for a drink of whisky. Now, if these people were really thirsty, or, in other words, if Nature was really calling for fluids, pure water would be just what they would first seek for, and pure water would be the thing which would best gratify the thirst. But, no! Water will not satisfy this soda-water or whisky thirst. Why? Simply because it is a craving of an appetite which is not a natural thirst, but which is, on the contrary, an abnormal appetite—a perverted taste. The appetite has been created—the habit acquired—and it is asserting the mastery.

A man acquires an appetite for tobacco in any of its forms; or for liquor, or for chewing-gum, or for opium, morphine, cocaine, or similar drugs. And an appetite once acquired becomes, if anything, stronger than that natural demand for food or drink, for men have been known to die of starvation because they had spent all of their money for drink or narcotics. Men have sold their babies' stockings for drink—have stolen and even murdered in order to gratify their appetite for narcotics. Who would think of calling this terrible craving of appetite by the name of Hunger? And yet we continue to speak and think of every craving for something to put into the stomach as Hunger, while many of these cravings are as much a symptom of Appetite as is the craving or desire for alcohol or narcotics.

The young child has a natural hunger until it is spoiled. In the child, natural hunger is more or less replaced by acquired appetites, the degree depending largely upon the amount of wealth its parents possess—the greater the wealth, the greater the acquirement of false appetite. And as it grows older, it loses all recollection of what real Hunger means. In fact, people speak of Hunger as a distressing thing, rather than as a natural instinct. Sometimes men go out camping, and the open air, exercise, and natural life gives them again a taste of real hunger, and they eat like school boys and with a relish they have not known for years. They feel 'hungry' in earnest, and eat because they have to, not from mere habit, as they do when they are home and are overloading their stomachs continually.

Natural hunger—like natural Thirst, expresses itself through the nerves of the mouth and throat. When one is hungry, the thought or mention of food causes a peculiar sensation in the mouth, throat and salivary glands. The saliva begins to flow, and the whole of the region manifests a desire to get to work. The stomach gives no symptoms whatever, and is not at all in evidence at such times. One feels that the 'taste' of good wholesome food would be most pleasurable. There is none of those feelings of faintness, emptiness, gnawing, 'all-gone-ness,' etc. in the region of the stomach. These last mentioned symptoms are all characteristic of the Appetite habit, which is insisting that the habit must be continued. Did you ever notice that the drink habit calls forth just such symptoms? The craving and 'all-gone' feeling is characteristic of both forms of abnormal appetite. The man who is craving a smoke or a chew of tobacco feels the same way.

A man often wonders why he cannot get a dinner such as 'mother used to cook.' He cannot get it simply because he has replaced his natural Hunger by an abnormal appetite, and he does not feel satisfied unless he gratifies that Appetite, which renders the homely fare of the past an impossibility. If the man were to cultivate a natural hunger, by a return to first principles, he would have restored to him the meals of his youth—he would find many cooks just as good as 'mother' was, for he would be a boy again.

You are probably wondering what all this has to do with Hatha Yoga. Well, just this: The Yogi has conquered appetite, and allows Hunger to manifest through him. He enjoys every mouthful of food, even to the crust of dry bread, and obtains nourishment and pleasure from it. He eats it in a manner unknown to most of you, he is a well-fed, properly nourished enjoyer of the feast, for he has possessed himself of that most piquant of all sauces—Hunger.

Food

WE intend to leave the matter of the choice of food an open question. While, personally, we prefer certain kinds of food, believing that the best results are obtained from the use thereof, we recognize the fact that it is impossible to change the habits of a lifetime (yes, of many generations) in a day, and man must be guided by his own experience and his growing knowledge, rather than by dogmatic utterances of others.

The Yogi theory of absorption of prana from food besides Nourishment holds that there is contained in the food of man and the lower animals, a certain form of prana which is absolutely necessary for man's maintenance of strength and energy, and that such form of prana is absorbed from the food by the nerves of the tongue, mouth and teeth. The act of mastication liberates this prana, by separating the particles of the food into minute bits, thus exposing as many atoms of prana to the tongue, mouth and teeth as possible. Once liberated from the food, this food-prana flies to the nerves of the tongue, mouth and teeth, passing through the flesh and bone readily, and is rapidly conveyed to numerous storage-houses of the nervous system, from whence it is conveyed to all parts of the body, where it is used to furnish energy and 'vitality' to the cells.

Now, let us consider Nature's plan in combining two important services in the act of masticating and salivating. In the first place, nature intended every particle of food to be thoroughly masticated and salivated before it was swallowed, and any neglect in this respect is sure to be followed by imperfect digestion. Insalivation of food is part of the digestive process, and certain work is done by the saliva which cannot be performed by the other digestive juices.

In the natural state of man, mastication was a most pleasant process, and so it is in the case of the lower animals, and the children of the human race to-day. The animal chews and munches his food with the greatest relish, and the child sucks, chews and holds in the mouth the food much longer than does the adult, until it begins to take lessons from its parents and acquires the custom of bolting its food. The Yogi theory is that while taste has much to do with it, still there is a something else, an indescribable sense of satisfaction obtained from holding the food in the mouth, rolling it around with the tongue, masticating it and allowing it to dissolve slowly and be swallowed almost unconsciously. While there remains a particle of taste in the food, nourishment is there to be extracted. But we believe that there is that other sensation which, when we allow it to manifest itself, gives us a certain satisfaction in the non-swallowing, and which sensation continues until all, or nearly all, the food-prana is extracted from the food. You will notice if you follow the Yogi plan of eating (even partially) that you will be reluctant to part with the food, and that, instead of bolting it at once, you will allow it to gradually melt away in the mouth until suddenly you realize that it is all gone. And this sensation is experienced from the plainest kinds of food, which do not appeal particularly to the taste, as well as to those foods which are special favourites of your particular taste.

When one has overcome the false Appetite (so often mistaken for Hunger) he will masticate a dry crust of whole-wheat bread and not only obtain a certain satisfaction of taste from the nourishment contained within it, but will enjoy the sensation of which we have spoken very keenly. The most nourishing of foods will yield the most satisfaction to the normal taste, and it is a fact to be remembered that food-prana is contained in food in direct proportion to its percentage of nourishment; another instance of Nature's wisdom.

The Yogi eats his food slowly, masticating each mouthful so long as he 'feels like it;' that is, so long as it yields him any satisfaction. In the majority of cases this sensation lasts so long as there remains any food in the mouth, as Nature's involuntary processes gradually causes the food to be slowly dissolved and swallowed. The Yogi moves his jaws slowly, and allows the tongue to caress the food, and the teeth to sink into it lovingly, knowing that he is extracting the food-prana from it, by means of the nerves of the mouth, tongue and teeth, and that he is being stimulated and strengthened, and that he is replenishing his reservoir of energy. At the same time he is conscious that he is preparing his food in the proper way for the digestive processes of the stomach and small intestines, and is giving his body good material needed for the building up of the physical body.

Those who follow the Yogi plan of eating will obtain a far greater amount of nourishment from their food than does the ordinary person, for every ounce is forced to yield up the maximum nourishment, while in the case of the man who bolts his food half-masticated and insufficiently insalivated, much goes to waste, and is passed from the system in the shape of a decaying, fermenting mass. Under the Yogi plan nothing is passed from the system as waste except the real waste matter, every particle of nourishment being extracted from the food, and the greater portion of the foodprana being absorbed from its atoms.

We understand fully that it is quite a different thing for the Yogi to take his time and eat in this manner and for the hurried man of business to do the same, and we do not expect all of our readers to change the habit of years all at once. But we feel sure that a little practice in this method of eating food will cause quite a change to come over one, and we know that such occasional practice will soon result in quite an improvement in the every-day method of masticating the food. We know, also, that the student will find a new delight—an additional relish in eating—and will soon learn to eat 'lovingly'. A new world of taste is opened up to the man who learns to follow this plan, and he will get far more pleasure from eating than ever before, and will have, besides, a much better digestion, and much more vitality, for he will obtain a greater degree of nourishment, and an increased amount of food-prana. It is possible for one who has the time and opportunity to follow this plan to its extreme limit, to obtain an almost unbelievable amount of nourishment and strength from a comparatively small amount of food. Those suffering from mal-nutrition and impaired vitality will find it profitable to at least partially follow this plan.

The Yogis prefer a non-animal diet, both from hygienic reasons and the aversion to eating the flesh of animals. The more advanced of the Yogi students prefer a diet of fruit, nuts, olive oil, etc. But when they travel among those who follow different dietary rules from themselves they do not hesitate to adapt themselves to the changed conditions, to a greater or less extent, and do not render themselves a burden to their hosts, knowing that if they follow the Yogi plan of masticating their food slowly their stomachs will take good care of what they eat.

We suggest that our readers consider whether or not they are eating too much meat; whether they are living upon too much fat and grease; whether they are eating enough fruit; whether they are not indulging in too much pastry and 'made dishes.' If we were asked to give them a general rule regarding eating we would be apt to say:

"Eat a variety of foods; avoid 'rich' dishes; do not eat too much fat; beware of the frying-pan; do not eat too much meat; avoid, especially, pig meat and veal; let your general habit of eating tend toward the simple, plain fare, rather than towards the elaborate dishes; go slow on pastry; masticate thoroughly and slowly; don't be afraid of food, if you eat it properly it will not hurt you, providing you do not fear it."

Keep as close to nature as possible and let her plans be your standard of measurement. The strong, healthy man is not afraid of his food, and neither should be the man who wishes to be healthy. Keep cheerful, breathe properly, eat properly, live properly, and you will not have occasion to make a chemical analysis of every mouthful of food. Do not be afraid to trust to your Instinct, for that is the natural man's guide, after all.

Water

ONE of the cardinal principles of the Hatha Yoga Philosophy of Health is the intelligent use of Nature's great gift to living things—Water. It should not be necessary to call the attention of men to the fact that Water is one of the great means of maintaining normal health, but man has become so much a slave to artificial environments, habits and customs, that he has forgotten Nature's laws. His only hope is to return to Nature.

The little child knows, instinctively, the use of water, and insists upon being furnished with it, but as it grows older it gets away from the natural habit, and falls into the erroneous practices of the older people around it. This is particularly true of those living in large cities, where the warm water drawn from taps is undrinkable, and so gradually become weaned away from the normal use of fluids. Such persons gradually form new habits of drinking (or not drinking), and, putting off nature's demands, they at last are not conscious of them. We often hear people say, "But why should we drink water—we do not get thirsty?" But had they continued in Nature's paths they would get thirsty, and the only reason why they do not hear Nature's calls is because they have so long turned a deaf ear to her that she has become discouraged and cries less loudly, besides their ears have ceased to recognize the vibrations, being so much taken with other things. Let man go back to Nature, and he will see water-drinking all around him, in all forms of life, from the plant up to the highest mammal. Who would think of depriving a plant of water? And who would be so cruel as to fail to provide the faithful horse with the requisite amount of water? And yet, man, while giving the plant and the animal that which his common sense teaches him they require, will deprive himself of the life-giving fluid, and will suffer the consequences.

So much importance does the Yogi attach to the proper use of drinking water, that he considers it one of the first principles of health. Water plays a most important part in the everyday life of the Hatha Yogi. He uses it internally and externally. He uses it to keep healthy, and he teaches its value to bring about healthy conditions, where disease has impaired the natural functioning of the body.

Let us see what water is used for in the body, and then make up our minds whether or not we have been living normal lives in this respect. In the first place, about seventy percent of our physical body is water! A certain amount of this water is being used up by our system, and leaves the body, constantly, and every ounce that is used up must be replaced by another ounce if the body is to be kept in a normal condition. The system is continuously excreting water through the pores of the skin, in the shape of sweat and perspiration. Sweat is the term applied to such excretion when it is thrown off so rapidly that it gathers and collects in drops. Perspiration is the term applied when the water is continuously and unconsciously evaporated from the skin. Experiments have shown that when perspiration is prevented the animal dies. Sweat and perspiration are shown by chemical analysis to be loaded with the waste products of the system—which, without a sufficient supply of fluids in the system, would remain in the body, poisoning it and bringing disease and death as a consequence. The repair work of the body is continually going on, the used-up and worn out tissue being carried off and replaced by fresh, new material from the blood, which has absorbed it from the nutrition in the food. If this waste matter is allowed to remain in the system it becomes a poison and breeds diseased conditions—it serves as a breeding place and all the rest of that family. Germs do not bother the clean and healthy system to any great extent, but let them come around one of these water-haters, and it finds his or her body full of uncast-off refuse and filth, and they settle down to business.

Both Perspiration and sweat are necessary, also, to dissipate the excessive bodily heat by their evaporation and thus keep down the bodily temperature to a normal degree. The perspiration and sweat also assist in carrying off the waste products of the system,—the skin being, in fact, a supplementary organ to the kidneys. Quite a quantity of water is exhaled through the lungs. The urinary organs pass off a large quantity, in performing their functions; about one and a half liter in twenty-four hours being the amount voided by the normal adult.

And all this has to be replenished, in order to keep the physical machinery going right. Water is also used by the body as a common carrier. It flows through the arteries and veins, and conveys the blood corpuscles and elements of nutrition to the various of the body, that they may be used in the building up process, which we have described. Without fluids in the system, the quantity of blood must decrease. On the return trip of the blood through the veins, the fluids take up the waste matter, and carry it to the excretory organism of the kidneys, the pores of the skin, and lungs, where the poisonous dead material and waste of the system is thrown off. Without sufficient fluids this work cannot be accomplished as Nature intended. And without sufficient water the waste portions of the food—cannot be kept sufficiently moist to easily pass through the colon and out of the body, and Constipation, with all of its attendant evils, result.

Every cell, tissue and organ needs water in order to be healthy. Water is a universal solvent and enables the system to assimilate and distribute the nourishment obtained from the food, and to get rid of the waste products of the system. It is often said that the "blood is the life," and if this is so, what must the water be called—for without water the blood would be but dust. Water is needed also for the purpose of enabling the kidneys to perform their functions of carrying off the urea, etc. It is needed in order to be manufactured into saliva, bile, pancreatic juice, gastric juices, and all the other valuable juices of the system, without which digestion would be impossible.

Now, how much water is needed to renew this waste? The best authorities agree that from two to two-and-a-half liter of water is the amount necessary to be taken daily by the average, normal man and woman, in order to make up the waste. If that amount is not supplied to the body it will withdraw fluids from the system until the person assumes that 'dried-up' look, with the consequence that all the physical functions are impaired, the person being 'dried-up' inside as well as on the surface.

The Yogis are not afraid to drink a sufficient amount of water each day. They are not afraid of 'thinning the blood,' as are some of these 'dried-up' people. Nature throws off the surplus quantity, if it be taken, very readily and rapidly. They do not crave 'ice water'—an unnatural product of civilization. Their favourite temperature is about room temperature. They drink when they are thirsty—and they have a normal thirst which does not have to be restored as does that of the 'dried-up' people. They drink frequently, but do not drink large quantities at any one time. They do not 'pour the water down,' believing that such a practice is abnormal and unnatural, and injurious. They drink it in small quantities, though often during the day. When working they often keep a vessel of water near them, and frequently sip there from.

The Yogis drink a cupful of water the last thing before going to bed at night. This is taken up by the system and is used in cleansing the body during the night, the waste products being excreted with the urine in the morning. They also drink a cupful immediately after arising in the morning; the theory being that by taking the water before eating it cleanses the stomach and washes away the sediment and waste which have settled during the night. They usually drink a cupful about an hour before each meal, following it by some mild exercise, believing that this prepares the digestive apparatus for the meal, and promotes natural hunger. They are not afraid of drinking a little water even at meals, but are careful not to 'wash-down' their food. Washing down the food with water not only dilutes the saliva, but causes one to swallow his food imperfectly insalivated and masticated, going down before Nature is ready. The Yogis believe that only in this way is water harmful when taken at meals. They take a little at each meal to soften up the food mass in the stomach, and that little does not weaken the strength of the gastric-juices, etc.

Many of our readers are familiar with the use of hot water as a means of cleansing a foul stomach. We approve of its use in that way, when needed, but we think that if our students will carefully follow the Yogi plan of living, as given in this book, they will have no foul stomachs needing cleansing—their stomachs will be good, healthy ones. As a preliminary toward rational eating, the sufferer may find it advantageous to use hot water in this way. The best way is to take about half a liter, slowly sipping it, in the morning before breakfast, or about one hour before other meals. It will excite a muscular action in the digestive organs, which will tend to pass from the system the foul matter stored there, which the hot water has loosened up and diluted, as well. But this is only a temporary expedient. Nature did not contemplate hot water as steady beverage, and water at ordinary temperature is all that she requires in health and that she requires to maintain health.

In addition to the properties, offices and uses of water, as above given, we will add that water contains prana in considerable quantities, a portion of which it parts with in the system, particularly if the system demands it. You all remember how at times a cup of cool water has acted as a powerful stimulant and 'refresher' to you, and how it enabled you to return to your work with renewed vigor and energy. Do not forget Water when you feel 'used up.' Used in connection with Yogi Breathing it will give a man fresh energy quicker than will any other method. In sipping water, let it remain in the mouth a moment before swallowing. The nerves of the tongue and mouth are the first (and quickest) to absorb the prana, and this plan will prove advantageous, particularly when one is tired. This is worth remembering.

Those who have neglected their natural instincts for many years have almost forgotten the natural habit of water drinking, and need considerable practice to regain it. A little practice will soon begin to create a demand for water, and you will in time regain the natural thirst. A good plan is to keep a glass of water near you, and take an occasional sip from it, thinking at the same time what you are taking it for. Say to yourself:

"I am giving my body the fluids it requires to do its work properly, and it will respond by bringing normal conditions back to me—giving me good health and strength, and making me a strong, healthy, natural human."

Fresh Air

NOW, do not pass-by this chapter, because it treats of a very common subject. If you feel inclined to so pass it by—then you are the very person for whom it is intended, and by whom it is most needed. This chapter is not intended to take up the subject of breathing, but will merely give a little preachment upon the necessity of fresh air and plenty of it— much needed by people where hermetically closed sleeping rooms, and air-tight houses are so much in vogue. We will come upon the subject of the importance of correct breathing, but the lesson will do you but little good unless you have good fresh air to breathe. Let us take a plain, common-sense, brief look at this subject.

You will remember that the lungs are constantly throwing off the waste matter of the system—the breath is being used as a scavenger of the body, carrying off the Waste products, broken down and refuse matter from all parts of the system. The matter thrown off by the lungs is almost as foul as that thrown off by the skin, the kidneys and even the bowels—in fact, if the supply of water given the system is not sufficient, nature makes the lungs do much of the work of the kidneys, in getting rid of the foul poisonous waste products of the body. And if the bowels are not carrying off the normal amount of waste matter, much of the contents of the colon gradually works through the system, seeking an outlet, and is taken up by the lungs and thrown off in the exhaled breath. Just think of it—if you shut yourself up in a tightly closed room, you are pouring out into the atmosphere of that room over thirty litres an hour of carbon dioxide, and other foul and poisonous gases. In eight hours you throw two-hundred and fifty litres. If there are two sleeping in the room, multiply the litres by two. As the air becomes contaminated, you breathe this poisonous matter over and over again into your system, the quality of the air becoming worse with each exhaled breath. No wonder that anyone coming into your room in the morning notices the stench pervading it, if you have kept the windows closed. No wonder you feel cross, stupid, quarrelsome, and generally 'grouchy' after a night in this kind of environment.

Did you ever think just why you sleep at all? It is to give nature a chance to repair the waste that has been going on during the day. You cease using up her energies in work, and give her a chance to repair and build up your system so that you will be all right the following day. And in order to do this work right, she requires at least normal conditions. She expects to be supplied with air containing the proper proportion of oxygen—air that has been exposed to the sunlight of the preceding day and which has thereby been freshly charged with prana. Any room that smells of that peculiar fetid odour that you have all noticed in a poorly ventilated bedroom, is no place for you to sleep in until it has been ventilated and kept supplied with fresh air. The air in a bedroom should be as nearly as possible kept as pure as the outside air. Don't be afraid of catching cold. Put on plenty of bed covering, and you will not mind the cold after you get a little used to it. Get back to nature! Fresh air does not mean sleeping in a draught, remember. And what is true of sleeping rooms is also true of living rooms, offices, etc. Of course, in winter one may not allow too much of the outside air to get into the house, as that would bring down the temperature too low, but still there is a happy compromise which may be made even in cold climates. Open the windows once in a while and give the air a chance to circulate in and out—so freshen things up a little, once in a while. Read up something on ventilation, and your health will be better. But even if you do not care to go that deep into the matter, think a little bit of what we have said, and your common sense will do the rest.

Get out awhile every day and let the fresh air blow upon you. It is full of life and health giving properties. You all know this, and have known it all your lives. But, nevertheless, you stick indoors in a manner which is entirely foreign to Nature's plans. No wonder you do not feel well. One cannot violate nature's rules with impunity. Do not be afraid of the air. Nature intended you to use it—it is adapted to your nature and requirements. So don't be afraid of it—learn to love it. Say to yourself while walking out and enjoying the fresh air:

"I am a child of Nature—she gives me this pure good air to use, in order that I may grow strong and well, and keep so. I am breathing in health and strength and energy. I am enjoying the sensation of the air blowing upon me, and I feel its beneficial effects. I am Nature's child, and I enjoy her gifts."

Learn to enjoy the air, and you will be blessed.

The Science of Breath

BREATHING may be considered the most important of all of the functions of the body, for, indeed, all the other functions depend upon it. Man may exist some time without eating; a shorter time without drinking; but without breathing his existence may be measured by a few minutes. To breathe is to live, and without breath there is no life.

"Breath is Life."

And not only is Man dependent upon Breath for life, but he is largely dependent upon correct habits of breathing for continued vitality and freedom from disease. An intelligent control of our breathing power will lengthen our days upon earth by giving us increased vitality and powers of resistance. Man in his normal state had no need of instruction in breathing. Like the lower animal and the child, he breathed naturally and properly, as nature intended him to do, but civilization has changed him in this and other respects. He has contracted improper methods and attitudes of walking, standing and sitting, which have robbed him of natural and correct breathing. He has paid a high price for civilization. The savage, today, breathes naturally, unless he has been contaminated by the habits of civilized man.

Physical health depends very materially upon correct breathing. In addition to the physical benefit derived from correct habits of breathing, man's mental power, happiness, self-control, clear-sightedness, morals, and even his spiritual growth may be increased by an understanding of the 'Science of Breath.' Whole schools of Oriental Philosophy have been founded upon this science.

Yogi Breathing

ONE of the first lessons in the Yogi Science of Breath is to learn how to breathe through the nostrils, and to overcome the common practice of mouth breathing. The organs of respiration have their only protective apparatus, filter, or dust catcher, in the nostrils. The nostrils are two narrow, tortuous channels, containing numerous bristly hairs which serve the purpose of a filter or sieve to strain the air of its impurities. The impurities that are stopped and retained by the sieves and mucous membrane of the nostrils are expelled when the breath is exhaled, and in case they have accumulated too rapidly or have managed to escape through the sieves and have penetrated forbidden regions, nature protects us by producing a sneeze, which violently ejects the intruder. Not only do the nostrils serve this important purpose, but they also perform an important function in warming the air inhaled. The long narrow winding nostrils are filled with warm mucous membrane, which coming in contact with the inhaled air warms it so that it can do no damage to the delicate organs of the throat, or to the lungs.

When the breath is taken through the mouth, there is nothing from mouth to lungs to strain the dust and other foreign matter in the air. And, moreover, such incorrect breathing admits cold air to the organs, thereby injuring them. Inflammation of the respiratory organs often results from the inhalation of cold air through the mouth.

The refining, filtering and straining apparatus of the nostrils renders the air fit to reach the delicate organs of the throat and lungs, and the air is not fit to reach these organs until it has passed through nature's refining process. We urge upon the student the necessity of acquiring this method of breathing if he has it not, and caution him against dismissing this phase of the subject as unimportant.

The Yogi knows all that his scientific brother knows about the physiological effect of correct breathing, but he also knows that the air contains more than oxygen and hydrogen and nitrogen, He knows something about prana, and he is fully aware of the nature and manner of handling that great principle of energy, and is fully informed as to its effect upon the human body and mind. He knows that by rhythmical breathing one may bring himself into harmonious vibration with Nature, and aid in the unfoldment of his latent powers. He knows that by controlled breathing he may not only cure disease in himself and others, but also practically do away with fear and worry and the baser emotions.

The Yogis classify Respiration into four general methods; High Breathing, Mid Breathing, Low Breathing and Yogi Complete Breathing. We will give a general idea of the first three methods, and a more extended treatment of the fourth method, upon which the Yogi Science of Breath is largely based.

High Breathing

THIS form of breathing is also known as Cavicular Breathing, or Collarbone Breathing. One breathing in this way elevates the ribs and raises the collarbone and shoulders, at the same time drawing in the abdomen and pushing its contents up against the diaphragm, which in turn is raised. The upper part of the chest and lungs, which is the smallest, is used, and consequently but a minimum amount of air enters the lungs. In addition to this, the diaphragm being raised, there can be no expansion in that direction. A maximum amount of effort is used to obtain a minimum amount of benefit.

Mid Breathing

THIS method of respiration is also known as Rib Breathing, or Inter-Costal Breathing, and while less objectionable than High Breathing, is far inferior to either Low Breathing or to the Yogi Complete Breath. In Mid Breathing the diaphragm is pushed upward, and the abdomen drawn in. The ribs are raised somewhat, and the chest is partially expanded. It is quite common among men who have made no study of the subject. As there are two better methods known, we give it only passing notice, to call your attention to its shortcomings.

Low Breathing

THIS form of respiration is far better than either of the two preceding forms, many writers have enthusiastically praised its merits, and have exploited it under the names of 'Abdominal Breathing,' 'Deep Breathing,' 'Diaphragmic Breathing,' etc. The diaphragm is the great partition muscle, which separates the chest and its contents from the abdomen and its contents. When at rest it presents a concave surface to the abdomen.—like a hill. When the diaphragm is brought into use the hill formation is lowered and the diaphragm presses upon the abdominal organs and forces out the abdomen. In Low Breathing, the lungs are given freer play than in the methods already mentioned, and consequently more air is inhaled.

Yogi Complete Breathing

DIRGHA PRĂNĂYĂMA,' or 'Yogi Complete Breathing' includes all the good points of High-, Mid- and Low Breathing, with the objectionable features of each eliminated. It brings into play the entire respiratory apparatus, every part of the lungs, every air-cell, and every respiratory muscle. The entire respiratory organism responds to this method of breathing, and the maximum amount of benefit is derived from the minimum expenditure of energy. The chest cavity is increased to its normal limits in all directions and every part of the machinery performs its natural work and functions.

One of the most important features of this method of breathing is the fact that the respiratory muscles are fully called into play. In Complete Breathing, among other muscles, those controlling the ribs are actively used, which increases the space in which the lungs may expand, and also gives the proper support to the organs when needed. Certain muscles hold the lower ribs firmly in position, while other muscles bend them outward. In this rib-action, the lower ribs are controlled by the diaphragm which draws them slightly downward, while other muscles hold them in place and the intercostal muscles force them outward, which combined action increases the mid-chest cavity to its maximum. In addition to this muscular action, the upper ribs are also lifted and forced outward by the intercostal muscles, which increases the capacity of the upper chest to its fullest extent.

The Yogi Complete Breath is the fundamental breath of the entire Yogi Science of Breath, and the student must fully acquaint himself with it, and master it perfectly before he can hope to obtain results from the other forms of breath mentioned. He should not be content with half-learning it, but should go to work in earnest until it becomes his natural method of breathing.

This Complete Breath is going back to first principles—a return to Nature. The healthy adult savage and the healthy infant of civilization both breathe in this manner, but civilized man has adopted unnatural methods of living, clothing and etcetera. The Complete Breath does not necessarily call for the complete filling of the lungs at every inhalation. One may inhale the average amount of air, using the Complete Breathing Method and distributing the air inhaled, be the quantity large or small, to all parts of the lungs. But one should inhale a series of full Complete Breaths several times a day, whenever opportunity offers, in order to keep the system in good order and condition. The following simple exercise will give you a clear idea of what the Yogi Complete Breath is:

I - Stand or sit erect. Breathing through the nostrils, inhale steadily, first filling the lower part of the lungs, which is accomplished by using the diaphragm, which descending exerts a gentle pressure on the abdominal organs, pushing forward the front walls of the abdomen.

II - Then fill the middle part of the lungs, pushing out the lower ribs, breastbone and chest.

III - Then fill the higher portion of the lungs, protruding the upper chest, thus lifting the chest, including the upper six or seven pairs of ribs. In the final movement, the lower part of the abdomen will be slightly drawn in, which movement gives the lungs a support and helps to fill the highest part of the lungs.

At first reading it may appear that this breath consists of three distinct movements. This, however, is not the correct idea. The inhalation is continuous, the entire chest cavity from the lowered diaphragm to the highest point of the chest in the region of the collarbone, being expanded with a uniform movement. Avoid a jerky series of inhalations, and strive to attain a steady continuous action. Practice will soon overcome the tendency to divide the inhalation into three movements, and will result in a uniform continuous breath. You will be able to complete the inhalation in a couple of seconds after a little practice.

IV - Retain the breath a few seconds.

V - Exhale quite slowly, holding the chest in a firm position, and drawing the abdomen in a little and lifting it upward slowly as the air leaves the lungs.

VI - When the air is entirely exhaled, relax the chest and abdomen. A little practice will render this part of the exercise easy, and the movement once acquired will be afterwards performed almost automatically.

By this method of breathing all parts of the respiratory apparatus are brought into action, and all parts of the lungs, including the most remote air cells, are exercised. The chest cavity is expanded in all directions. You will also see that the Complete Breath is really a combination of Low, Mid and High Breaths, succeeding each other rapidly in the order given, in such a manner as to form one uniform, continuous, complete breath.

Yogi Complete Breath Exercises

THESE breathing exercises while utilizing the Yogi Complete Breath are very good in their own right in helping to build a proper habit of breathing, but also before commencing physical exercises and yoga postures. The exercises activate all the portions of your lungs and air-cells and warm up the muscles of the respiratory system in preparation for the practice that follows.

Hands In-and Out Breathing

STAND erect with your arms stretched in front of you. Inhale a full Yogi Complete Breath while you move your arms to the sides keeping them horizontal and level with the ground. Exhale while moving your arms back to the front, always keeping your arms straight. Repeat a couple of full yogi breaths.

Hand Stretch Breathing

STAND straight, interlock your fingers and place your hands on your chest. Now while inhaling a full Yogi Complete Breath stretch your arms straight in front of you, pushing your palms to the front. Then exhale and move your palms back on your chest. Relax the arms and shoulders. Repeat this movement for a couple of full yogi breaths and then move the stretching of your arms a little up to the forehead level. After a few more breaths on this level, stretch your arms straight up, pushing the palms up, always keeping the fingers interlocked. Again, repeat this upward stretching for a few complete yogi breaths. Then end the exercise by releasing your hands and relaxing your shoulders.

Ankle Stretch Breathing

STAND straight with your arms by the sides of the body. While you inhale a Complete Yogi Breath, you move your stretched arms straight up from your front side, while lifting your heels off the ground so that you stand on your toes. Exhale and move your arms down while standing your heels back down on the floor. Repeat a few complete yogi breaths.

Physical Exercise

MAN in his original state did not need to be instructed in physical exercise—neither does a child or youth with normal tastes. Man's original state of living gave him an abundance of varied activities, out-of-doors, and with all the best conditions for exercise. He was compelled to seek his food, to prepare it, to raise his crops, to build his houses, to gather up fuel, and to do the thousand and one things which were necessary to live in simple comfort. But as man began to be civilized he also began to delegate certain of his duties to others, and to confine himself to one set of activities, until at the present day many of us do practically no physical work, while others do nothing but hard physical labour of a limited scope—both living unnatural lives.

Physical labour without mental activity dwarfs a man's life—and mental labour without some sort of physical activity also dwarfs the man's life. Nature demands the maintaining of the balance—the adoption of the happy medium. The natural, normal life calls for the use of all of man's powers, mental and physical, and the man who is able to so regulate his life that he gets both mental and physical exercise is likely to be the healthiest and happiest.

The Yogis believe that the instinct toward games—the feeling that exercise is needed, is but the same instinct that causes man to labour at congenial occupations—it is the call of nature toward activity—varied activity. The normal, healthy body is a body that is equally well nourished in all of its parts, and no part is properly nourished unless it is used. A part that is unused receives less than the normal amount of nourishment and in time becomes weakened. Nature has provided man with exercise for every muscle and part of his body, in natural work and play. By natural work, we do not mean the work attendant upon some particular form of bodily labour, for a man following one trade only exercises one set of muscles, and is likely to become 'muscle-bound,' and is in as much need of exercise as the man who sits at his desk all day, with the exception that the man working at his trade usually has the advantage of more out-of- door life.

We consider the modern plans of 'Physical Culture' very poor substitutes for out-of-door work and play. They have no interest attached to them, and the mind is not called to participate as is in the case of work or games. But still anything in the way of exercise is better than nothing. But we protest against that form of Physical Culture which has for its object the enlargement of certain muscles, and the performance of the feats of the 'strong men.' All this is unnatural. The perfect system of physical culture is that one which tends to produce a uniform development of the entire body—the employment of all the muscles—the nourishment of every part and which adds as much interest as possible to the exercise, and which keeps its practitioners out in the open air.

The Yogi allows his exercise to call into operation his mind. He takes an interest in the exercises, and by an effort of the will sends an increased flow of prana to the part brought into motion. He thus obtains a multiplied benefit, and a few minutes exercise do him as much good as would ten times that amount of exercise, if performed in the usual indifferent, uninterested way. This 'knack' of sending the mind to the desired part is easily acquired. All that is necessary is to accept as a fact the statement that it can be done, thus doing away with all subconscious resistance, caused by the doubting mental attitude; then simply command the mind to send a supply of prana to the part, and to increase the circulation there. The mind does this to a certain extent involuntarily, the moment that the attention is centred on a part of the body, but the effect is greatly increased by the effort of the Will. The simplest way to accomplish the desired result is to confidently expect that what you wish will happen. This 'confident expectation' acts practically as a strong and positive command of the Will—put it into operation and the thing is accomplished.

For instance, if you wish to send an increased amount of prana to the forearm, and to increase the circulation to that part, thereby increasing the nourishment, simply double the arm, and then gradually extend it, fastening the gaze or attention upon the lower arm, and holding the thought of the desired result. Do this several times, and you will feel that the forearm has been greatly exercised, although you have used no violent motion, and have used no apparatus. Try this plan on several parts of the body, making some muscular motion in order to get the attention there, and you will soon acquire the skill, so that when you go through any ordinary simple exercise you will do this almost automatically. In short, when you exercise, realize what you are doing and what you are doing it for, and you will get the result. Put life and interest into your exercise, and avoid the listless, mechanical manner of going through the motions, so common in physical culture exercises. Put some 'fun' into it, and enjoy it. Carry the thought of 'strength and development' with you while you exercise, and you will get much better results. In this way both mind and body obtain a benefit, and you will leave your exercise with a splendid glow and thrill such as you have not experienced for many a day.

As general advice before commencing any physical exercise, it is best to always perform the exercise when the stomach is empty. Nor should force or pressure be used; the body should not tremble while you practice. Perform any posture to the limits of your abilities and never beyond. Always lower the head and other parts of the body slowly and breathe with control. The benefits increase if the specific breathing technique to the ăsana is performed. Over time you will improve and nothing will be able to stop you from becoming as healthy, strong and flexible as you can be, provided you listen to your body and practice faithfully. Lastly, if your body is stressed, you feel a little tired or have an elevated heartbeat, rest in Savăsana (corpse pose). Other good ăsanas for rest are; after inverted ăsanas, Balăsana (child pose); following postures lying on the abdomen use Makarăsana (crocodile pose) and after standing exercises, Tadăsana (mountain pose). The details as to how to perform these and other ăsanas you will find under their corresponding chapters.

In the following chapter you will find some loosening exercises (Sithilĭkarana Vyăyăma), and further on, Ăsanas. Followed faithfully, these will give you all the movements necessary to exercise your entire body, bringing every part into action, strengthening every organ, and making you not only well developed, but also straight and erect, and as supple and quick of movement as an athlete. It is just the thing you have been looking for, with all the unnecessary features 'trimmed off.' Try the exercises for a while, before you make up your mind about them. They will practically 'make you over' physically, if you will but take the time and trouble to put them into faithful practice.

In the last section of this book there is offered a suggested exercise plan. This plan combines exercises to be found throughout this work into a program that will address your whole body in a most effective way.

Sithilikarana Vyăyăma

LOOSENING EXERCISES' or Sithilikarana Vyăyăma are normally performed with some speed and repetitions. They not only help in performing yogăsanas (yoga postures) better by loosening the joints, but they also help in building up stamina and tolerance.

These few exercises will faithfully address all the joints that can be manipulated in your body. Repeat each individual movement of every exercise for a fair amount of repetitions to have the most out of them. It is better to start with a few repetitions of any exercise at first, and then gradually increase the number. There is no harm in prolonging these exercises so long as it is without strain or fatiguing yourself.

Chest, back and shoulder loosening

I- Extend the arms straight out in front of you, on the level of the shoulder, with palms of the hands touching each other. (2) Swing back the hands until the arms stand out straight, sideways from the shoulders, or even a little further back if they will go there easily without forcing; return briskly to your starting position and repeat several times. It is an improvement if you rise on your toes during the backward sweep, sinking on your heels as you move the arms forward again.

II- Extend the arms straight out from the shoulder, sideways, with opened hands; (2) With the arms so extended, swing the hands around in circles, (not too wide) keeping the arms back as far as possible, and not allowing the hands to pass in front of the line of the breast while making the circles

Hips and Knees Loosening

I - Inhale while standing erect. With knees far apart, but heels almost touching each other, sit down while exhaling. Balance on the toes and sit on the heels. (2) Try to push the knees apart by the palms and breathe in while getting up.

II - Stand erect with hands straight down. Inhale completely, then breathe out while going down by bending the knee-joints and keeping them together. Keep the body straight without bending at the waist and inhale while you come up.

Ankles and toes Loosening

I - Sit with your legs straight in front of you, and the hands resting in your lap. Look at your toes and spread them as wide as possible. Then contract your toes and bend them down as strong as you can. Repeat a few times. (2) Then wiggle each toe individually one after the other. This may prove impossible but in time, your capability to do so will increase steadily. Remember to look at each toe that you intent to move enforcing the movement of each individual toe by your will.

II - Move both feet back and forth, bending from the ankle and stretch the feet forward to touch the floor if you can. Ten draw them back towards the knees, holding each position for a few seconds. Do not bend your knees!

III - Rotate each foot separately clockwise and anticlockwise ten times, and then rotate both feet together simultaneously first in one, than in the other direction. Finally rotate the feet simultaneously, but each in opposite directions.

IV - Fold the right foot on the left thigh. Grab your right foot with your left hand, your right calf with your right. Then rotate your ankle numerous times using only your hand, relaxing the ankle completely. Do the same in the other direction, then repeat with the other leg folded.

Knees Loosening and Hip Rotation

I - Sit with your legs straight in front of you, and the hands resting in your lap. Bend the right knee and hold your right thigh with both hands. Then straighten the right leg and straighten your arms, then bend your leg and move your thigh close to the chest with the heel near the buttocks. Keep your head and spine straight while moving your leg back and forth. Do the same with the other knee bent.

II - Place one foot on the opposite thigh and hold the bent knee with the corresponding hand. Rotate the knee clockwise and then anticlockwise using the arm to make big circles. (2) Now straighten your leg. Bend it once, bringing the right heel near the buttock. Then straighten the leg again. Now exercise the other leg the same way.

III - Stretch your legs in front of you and place your hands under the buttocks. First move your right leg at the hip joint, describing a circle clockwise for five to ten times. The knee bends as the circle reaches the chest, and the leg stretches as the foot reaches its farthest point from your body. Then repeat the same with the other leg.

Perform the next exercises while you are sitting down on your knees with the buttocks resting on the heels and the front of the feet flat on the floor and your hands resting in the lap. Alternatively, if your legs would allow it, you can sit with the buttocks between the feet on the floor.

Fingers Loosening

I - Sit on your heels. Stretch your arms straight in front of you hands touching each other with the palms down. Make fists and clench your hands. Then with force spread your fingers and push the fingers out. Keep your arms straight and repeat the clenching and stretching for a few times.

Wrists Loosening

II - Sit on your heels. Stretch your arms straight in front of you, grab your right wrist with your left hand, and then rotate your right hand five times clockwise and then anticlockwise. Repeat holding the other wrist. (2) Then release your grip and rotate both wrists simultaneously one clockwise and the other counter clockwise, and repeat the same reversing the direction of each wrist.

III - Stretch your arms straight in front of you hands touching each other with the palms down. Then bend your wrists down and stretch. Release and bend your wrists up, again stretch. Repeat alternating until you have done five stretches in each direction.

Elbows Loosening

I - Sit on your heels. Stretch your arms straight in front of you, then bend your left arm and support your elbow with your right hand. Rotate your upper left arm in big circles five times clockwise and then anticlockwise.

II - Keep hold of your elbow and straighten your arm with the palm facing down. Then turn your palm up, fold your arm and touch your shoulder with the hand repeatedly. Now do both exercises with the other arm.

Shoulders Loosening

I - Sit on your heels. Fold your arms and grab your shoulders. Rotate the elbows five times clockwise and then anticlockwise in as big a circles as you possibly can.

II - Keep a hold of the shoulders, and then while you exhale, move the elbows towards each other touching in front of the chest. Hold a few seconds and exhale slowly while moving the elbows to the sides. Repeat five times before releasing the hands.

Neck Loosening

Sit in a comfortable position and rest your hands on your lap, relax your body and let your shoulders drop; make sure they are not hunched and close your eyes. Each step describes one round, do each three to ten times.

I - Tilt the head forwards, return the head to the upright position and tilt the head backwards. Tilt the head forward again to the normal position. The whole movement is one smooth slow motion.

II - Bend the head to each side, with the ear going towards the shoulder in a smooth slow motion.

III - Rotate your head clockwise in as large a circle as possible. Ensure that the shoulders remain relaxed. Then repeat the same rotation anticlockwise.

Cross-legged Lumbarstretch

You start this exercise from the position where you are lying down on your back. Be flat on the floor with your legs together and straight, and the arms by the sides with the palms facing down. You will notice while practicing the stretch that the whole abdominal area, your hips and thighs come into play, especially the lumbar (lower back) muscles. The twisting of the spine will relieve the stiffness caused by sitting for long stretches of time, and lengthen your back muscles through its continued practice.

I - Lie down on the back with your legs together and the arms spread sideways at shoulder level, then bend your legs from the knees and place the soles flat on the floor.

II - Place your right leg over the left leg and lock the right foot behind the left calf. If you cannot reach than keep one leg crossed over the other. Inhale.

III - While you exhale, lower the knees to the right towards the floor, turn the head to the left and keep the shoulders touching on the floor. Breathe normal and remain in this position for a while.

IV - Inhale and bring the knees and the head back to the centre. Then exhale and lower the knees to the left side, the head to the right.

V - Repeat these steps twice, then on an exhale come back to centre, release your legs, cross and lock the left leg over the right. Now repeat the same sequence, again twice, stretching the other side.

Sŭrya Namaskăra

SUN SALUTATION' is a rhythmic and symmetric sequence of movements, a real pleasure to perform! It revitalizes the whole body, removes all signs of sleep and prepares your body and mind for the practice that follows. The benefits of ăsanas, mudras as well as pranayama can be attained through its use alone, maybe for when you have just a little time available. The Sŭrya Namaskăra can be practised at almost any time of the day and in any place. No special preparations are necessary. There is no reason why most people cannot practice it daily. It only takes a matter of ten minutes or so and during this short period of time the body is exercised in the most systematic and comprehensive manner possible. There is no other exercise that can surpass it.

It induces the inflow of pure vital air in sufficient quantities in the lungs, which makes the body glow like the sun. This exercise has twelve components. For each part of the body there is a provision of a separate and distinctive type of Sŭrya Namaskăra, so that not even the tiniest part of the body escapes its wholesome influence. A regular practice of this sequence of yoga postures will broaden the chest and strengthen your arms, shoulders, and abdominal muscles. It relieves constipation and stimulates digestion. Its practice makes the spine and waist flexible and will keep your whole body supple. If you practice this pose regularly it will help you to calm your mind and to improve your focus and concentration. This exercise is a complete workout! Patients of hernia are warned against its practice though, until they have sufficiently resolved the issue and strengthened the afflicted area.

It is very good to make the Sun Salutation a part of your daily yoga practice. Perform Sŭrya Namaskăra at sunrise and sunset since the exercise has a definite relationship to the sun and full advantage is derived by its being performed at the right time. There are twelve steps involved in performing Sŭrya Namaskăra. Each step is accompanied by a regulation of the breath. This can be done, facing the sun, after chanting the following verse:

Hiranmayena Pătrena Satyasyăpihitam Mukham, Tat tvam Pŭsan Apăvrnu Satya-dharmăya Drstaye

Like a lid to a vessel, O Sun, your Golden orb covers the entrance to Truth. Kindly open the entrance, to lead me to Truth.

The steps are as follows:

I - Stand straight with your legs together, your arms down and shoulders relaxed (Tădăsana.) Breathe normally and relax, then bring your palms together in front of your chest, forming the traditional Indian gesture for greeting, called 'Namaskăra'

II - Inhale and raise both arms above your head; bend the head, arms and upper trunk backwards with your palms facing forwards,

III - Exhale and bend forward, then place your palms on the floor next to the feet and (try to) touch the knees with your forehead or chin while keeping the legs straight,

IV - Inhale and stretch your right leg back while bending your left leg, but keeping the left foot and your palms in position. Keep your arms straight, arch your back and head upwards and look up.

V - Hold your breath and take your left leg back and place it next to your right, supporting yourself on your palms and toes only. Keep your arms straight, and the body straight, at an angle of about 30 degrees inclined to the ground.

VI - Exhale and bend your knees, keeping the hands and toes in position. Rest first the knees, then forehead and lastly your chest on the ground with your buttocks raised up.

VII - Inhale while you simultaneously lower the hips to the floor and straighten your arms. Arch your head and back upwards. Keep the position of the hands and feet but straighten your toes back.

VIII - Exhale and raise the buttocks to make an arch with your heels and palms touching the floor, the arms and knees straight, and pushing your head down.

IX - Inhale and bring your left leg in between your arms and place your foot flat on the floor, in line with the hands. Keep your right leg straight, arch the back and head upwards and look up.

X - Exhale and bring the right foot forward next to the left foot, keeping your palms on the floor next to the feet. Touch your knees with the forehead or chin and keep the legs straight.

XI - Inhale and come straight, taking your straight arms from the front to all the way above the head in a big circle, and bend your upright arms, head and back further backwards.

XII - Exhale, come straight and lower your hands along the body so you are standing back in the starting position, Tadăsana. Relax and breathe normally.

Sūrya Namaskăra
Sun Salutation

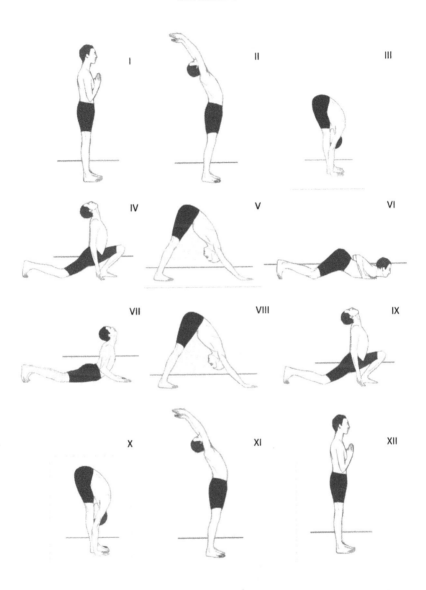

These twelve positions constitute a half round of Sŭrya Namaskăra. To complete the second half repeat the same positions, except in positions IV and IX where you reverse the order of the leg movements

While performing each step you can (mentally) chant the different names of the Sun and meditate on those qualities during the practice.

Om Hram Mitrăya Namah	*Greetings to the*...friend of all beings
Om Hrim Ravaye Namah	...shining
Om Hrum Suryaya Namah	...dispeller of darkness
Om Hraĭm Bhănave Namah	...one who illumines
Om Hroum Khagaya Namah	...one who is all-pervading
Om Hrah Pŭsne Namah	...nourishment fulfilment
Om Hram Hiranyagarbhăya Namah	...one with golden brilliance
Om Hrim Marĭcaye Namah	...light with infinite rays
Om Hrum Adityaya Namah	...son of Aditi (Divine Mother)
Om Hraĭm Savitre Namah	...one responsible for life
Om Hroum Arkăya Namah	...worthy of praise and glory
Om Hrar Bhăskarăya Namah	...wisdom and illumination

Ăsanas

POSTURES.' Yoga first originated in India, and the greatest classical text from the Yoga Philosophy is the Yoga Sutras by Patanjali. Patanjali describes ăsana as the third of the eight limbs of Raja Yoga. The eight limbs are, in order, the yamas—restrictions, niyamas—observances, ăsanas—postures, pranayama— breath work, pratyahara— sense withdrawal or non-attachment, dharana— concentration, dhyana— meditation, and samadhi—realization of the true Self or Atman.

Ăsanas are the physical aspect of Yoga. Patanjali suggests that the only requirement for practicing ăsanas is that it be "steady and comfortable." The body is held poised with the practitioner experiencing no discomfort. Ăsanas are to discipline the body, to keep it disease-free and for preserving vital energy. Correct postures are a physical aid to meditation, for they control the limbs and nervous system and prevent them from producing disturbances.

When you witness a Yogi skilled in ăsanas, you have the sense that his body is in continuous subtle motion. One feature distinguishing an asana from a stretch or gymnastic exercise is that in ăsana practice the Yogi mind is completely focused so that he may move as a whole and perceive what the body has to tell. In modern fast paced cultures this is rarely done. People watch TV while stretching; a book is read while walking the treadmill; a most common sight is a jogger or gymnast wearing headphones listening to a portable music device. Problems are mulled over in the mind while taking a walk or while doing any of the popular exercise programs that are the current hype. One keeps a constant watch over others to benchmark our own level of accomplishment.

The word ăsana is usually translated as 'pose' or 'posture,' but its more literal meaning is 'comfortable seat.' Through their observations of nature, the yogis discovered a vast repertoire of expressions that have strong physical effects on the body, and psychological effects to the mind. Each movement demands that we address some aspect of our consciousness and use ourselves in a new way. The Yogi believes that consciousness is present throughout every aspect of the body, and the diversity of ăsanas is no accident, for through exploring both familiar and unfamiliar postures we are expanding our consciousness. Sri Dharma Mittra (a Yoga teacher) suggested that *"there are an infinite number of ăsanas"*, when he first began to catalogue the number of ăsanas as an offering of devotion to his guru Swami Kailashananda Maharaj. He eventually compiled a list of 1300 variations, derived from contemporary gurus, yogis, and ancient and contemporary texts. This work is considered one of the primary references for ăsanas in the field of yoga today.

Tădăsana

MOUNTAIN POSE' is the first in the group of ăsanas that we will cover, as it is a starting position for many postures. This pose is good for the mental preparation of upcoming exercises and it will help you to focus and to calm the mind. Tădăsana makes you aware of how a healthy posture looks like and helps to keep a good stance throughout your daily life.

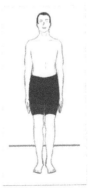

I- Stand straight with your feet parallel to each other. Put your arms next to your body, hanging them loose. Keep your knees straight, your head upright and the shoulders and body relaxed. Close your eyes and breathe normal.

II- Focus that you stand straight on both of your feet with the weight equally on both sides. Do not swing back and forth and keep your attention on your breathing, which will help to stand straight, to calm down and to concentrate on the upcoming yoga pose and the influences on your body of the preceding ăsana.

Trikonăsana

TRIANGLE POSE.' All the movements of Trikonăsana have a wonderful influence in the region of the waist and the entire nervous system is positively affected, especially the spinal nerves. This posture builds up strength in the lower back and upper legs while removing tension from the lower and upper back, the hips and the hamstrings through both the twist and the stretching. It loosens up the muscles and joints and revitalizes the whole body. The asana proves useful for patients of sciatica, if practiced slowly and without jerks. The Triangle Pose is good for your sense of coordination and balance, and you need concentration and precision to carry it out correctly. It is by keeping the body in this posture for some time that its advantages can be obtained in full.

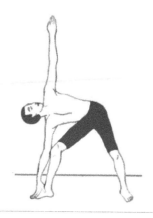

I- Stand erect with your feet about one meter apart. Inhale and extend your arms horizontally to each side.

II - Exhale and bend at the waist towards the right side so that your left arm points straight up and your right arm points down. Make sure your left palm is facing forward and look up at your left hand. Breathe normally.

III - Inhale and come up keeping your arms horizontally extended to each side.

IV - Exhale and bend to the left side so that your right arm points straight up and your left arm points down. Look up at your right hand which has the palm facing forward and breathe normally.

V - Inhale and come up keeping your arms horizontally to each side.

VI - Exhale and bring your legs together by moving one foot to the other, and bring your arms down from the sides, breathe normally and relax the shoulders.

A more advanced variation to this pose is called 'PSARIVRTTA TRIKONĀSANA,' 'Crossed Triangle pose.'

I - Stand straight with your feet about 1 meter apart. Inhale and extend your arms horizontally to each side.

II - Bend forward at the waist so that your head, trunk and arms lie in one horizontal plane. Look forwards. Exhale and Swivel your trunk to the right and touch your right foot with your left hand, right arm pointing upwards.

III - At the end of the movement, twist your head and look upwards at your right hand. This is the final position. Stay in the final position for a few seconds. Breathe normally.

IV - Inhale and swing your left arm back into the standing position with your arms horizontally to each side.

V - Bend forward. Exhale and Swivel your trunk to the left touch your left foot with your right hand, left arm pointing upwards. Look up at your left hand. Breathe normally.

VI - Inhale and swing your right arm back into the standing position with your arms horizontally to each side. Exhale, lower your arms and move feet together.

Părsvakonăsana

SIDE ANGLE POSE.' A special feature of the 'Părsvakonăsana is that it helps in increasing height. The asana makes the body well-proportioned and it becomes light. Practicing the side angle pose relieves backache and develops the buttocks. It proves useful for patients of sciatica, if practiced slowly. But it should not be performed in jerks or hastily for then it loses all its excellence and usefulness. It is only by keeping the body in this posture for some time that its advantages can be obtained. There are many other benefits that come from practicing this pose. It improves and strengthens the legs, knees, and ankles. Părsvakonăsana stretches the groin, waist and also the back from the twisting of the spine in the more advanced exercise. Staying balanced is very important for this asana, improving both your balance and stamina greatly.

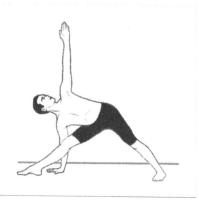

I - Stand straight with your feet about 1 meter apart. Inhale and extend your arms horizontally to each side.

II - Turn your left foot a little in to the right, and your right foot out to the right 90 degrees. Turn your right thigh outward, and the left hip slightly forward, but rotate your upper torso back to the left.

III - Move your left arm up, stretch towards the ceiling and then towards the right side from over your head while you bend your right knee directly over the ankle.

IV - Place your right palm on the floor to the side of your foot and look up at your left hand. Stay in this final pose for a comfortable length of time, breathing normally.

V- Inhale and return to the standing pose by reversing the steps. Then repeat the same, but turning towards the other side.

There are quite a few variations possible for this asana, and if you find the preceding exercise easy, you can try the challenging 'PARIVRTTA PĀRSVAKONĀSANA', the 'Revolved Side Angle Pose'.

I- Stand straight with your feet about 1 meter apart. Inhale and extend your arms horizontally to each side.

II- Turn your left foot a little in to the right, and your right foot out to the right 90 degrees. Turn your right thigh outward, and the left hip slightly forward.

III- Exhale and lean your torso downwards and turn it towards the right. Place your left hand on the floor, next to your right foot on the right side, leaning your upper body further towards the back. Turn your head towards the right and fix your gaze on the right hand. Stay in this final pose for a comfortable length of time, breathing normally.

IV- Inhale and return to the standing pose by reversing the steps. Then repeat the instructions, but turning towards the other side.

Natarăjăsana

LORD OF THE DANCE POSE.' Natarăjă,' which means 'Lord Of The Dance' is one of the names given to the Hindu God Shiva in his form as the cosmic dancer —Lord Sankara— and is regarded as the source of knowledge of yoga. The Natarăjăsana is so widely popular that many a representation of this asana can be found, composed in a variety of materials and in all sizes, from the smallest to the largest. Some use these for decoration of their homes, whereas others treat them as the images of Lord Sankara and, therefore, worship them. It is thus that Natarăjăsana comes to be the most widely known asana.

This is a balancing ăsana that strengthens the legs, stretches the whole body and develops concentration and grace, being considered the most charming in creation. For the practice of Natarăjăsana one foot is planted on the ground while the other is raised in various directions. One hand is kept on the forehead while the other is moved as required; the head is kept steady but the gaze is shifted in different directions. There are innumerable possibilities of the asana. In attempting to signify the different emotions appropriate expressions are assumed by the face, the eyes, and the limbs. It is believed that Lord Sankara, when dancing, assumes four arms, which is impossible for mortals. Yet, the practice of Natarăjăsana is an incomparable asset for dancers. Its practice develops awareness of the mysteries of the art of dancing and dexterity in the technique of the dance. It is generally conceded that on earth there is no one who can actually and properly perform this asana as Lord Sankara can.

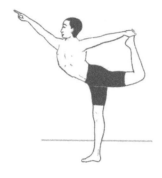

I - Stand straight. Bend your right leg and grab your ankle or big toe with the left hand.

II - Inhale, lift the right leg up, and bring the thigh parallel to the floor.

III - Reach the left arm straight forward, parallel to the floor. This is the final pose. Hold it for about 30 seconds, release, and repeat the other side.

Ardha Katicakrăsana

LATERAL ARC POSE.' Through 'Ardha Katicakrăsana, the lateral thoracic muscles are stretched and the elasticity of the spine increases. Hip joints become flexible and excess fat around the waist reduces.

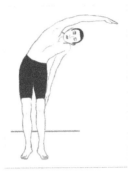

I - Stand straight with the feet a little apart. Relax the shoulders and keep the neck straight and palms stretched by the sides.

II - Inhale and slowly raise your right arm from the side up, at shoulder level turn your palm facing up, and keep raising your arm until your biceps touch the right ear, hand pointing up and palm facing left. Stretch up

III - Exhale and bend towards your left side from the waist. Keep your arms, legs and body in line. Breathe normally.

IV - Inhale and come up, back to the vertical position.

V - Exhale and slowly lower your arm down in a synchronized movement with the breath. At shoulder level turn your palm and continue until the arm is next to the body.

VI - Repeat with the left arm pointing up, bending to the right side. At the end of the complete ăsana, rotate and relax the shoulders

Pada Hastăsana

FORWARD BENDING POSE' is easy to perform, yet it is very beneficial. Even a little practice can produce an immediate and noticeable effect. This exercise is ideal for the resilience of the spine, strengthening and loosening it up, relocating minor displacements of vertebrae and releasing nerves that may be pinched, removing aches and pains in the back, neck and head. Simultaneously, it stretches and strengthens the backs of the legs, makes the shoulders strong, the chest broad, and the waist slim. Pada Hastăsana helps in reducing weight. Because the upper part of the body is turned upside down for most of the practice, blood circulation to the brain is stimulated, improving its efficiency.

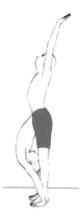

I - Stand erect. Place the feet together not touching each other. Let the arms relax and hang beside the body. Keep the legs straight throughout the practice. Inhale and move the arms up from the sides until the hands point upwards and stretch up.

II - Slowly exhale and bend the arms and body forwards, until your head and trunk point towards the floor.

III - Place your palms on the floor besides the feet and touch the knees with the head. Alternatively, you can grasp your ankles, big toes or put your hands under your feet with the palms up. In that case, use a slight stretching force with your arms to lengthen the body. Breathe normally and remain in this position for a minute or so, allowing the back muscles to stretch.

IV - Inhale and slowly raise the body and stretched arms to the erect position until the arms are stretched up above the head.

V - Exhale and lower your arms from the sides synchronizing your breath and movement. Relax and breathe normally, then repeat the exercise once more.

Ardha Chakrăsana

HALF WHEEL POSE.' Athough quite easy to perform, the 'Ardha Chakrăsana' has many advantages. The ribs acquire resilience whereby many respiratory ailments can be prevented. It is beneficial for your heart and can help to regulate high blood pressure. As it stretches your abdomen, abdominal organs and intestines, it helps your digestion making your inner organs work properly. The bending backwards will bring flexibility to your spine and hips while the shoulders, neck, arms, abdomen, back, and thighs are strengthened. It is equally useful for men as well as women.

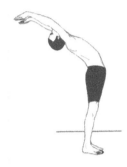

I - Stand straight. Keep your feet hip-width apart. Exhale and place your hands on your lower back just above your buttocks

II - With inhalation bend your head and back backwards as much as your body allows you. Stay in this position and keep breathing normally.

III - Come up with exhalation, release the hands and relax the arms hanging down from the shoulders. You can repeat the posture 3 to 5 times, and then relax the arms and shoulders.

Vrkṣāsana

TREE POSE' helps you practicing balance. Poor balance is often the result of a restless mind or distracted attention. Regular practice will help focus the mind and cultivate concentration (dharana) and coordination. Because the weight of the entire body is balanced on one foot, the muscles of that leg are strengthened. Imagine you are a tree, growing its roots deep into the earth, stretching its branches towards the sky.

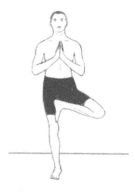

I - Stand straight, bring your right foot up with inhalation and place it on the inner side of your left thigh as high as it will go.

II - When you have found your balance, place your hands in front of your chest with the palms touching each other, and slowly bring them over your head, stretching up.

III - Keep your eyes on a fixed point in front of you, so you can balance better. This is the final pose. Breathe normally and stay thus for a minute or so.

IV - Then bring down your arms and leg and repeat the same exercise from the other side.

Garudăsana

EAGLE POSE.' Garuda is the mythical bird that transports Lord Vishnu (a Hindu god) throughout the celestial realms. The 'Garudăsana,' provides great strength to the feet and thighs, and is of special benefit to those who have to walk long distances. Its practice even for a short while after a journey on foot quickly relieves fatigue. Any ache or disorder of the knees, the feet, and other joints, as well as pain or tremulousness of the shoulders, the elbows, the arms, and the forearms, is remedied by the practice of this asana. The Eagle Pose helps to bring about mental and physical harmony. It also develops poise and grace in the body.

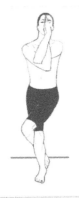

I- Take a standing position and breathe normally the whole practice. Raise the right leg and twist it around the left leg; the right thigh in front of the left thigh and the right foot rests on the calf of the left leg..

II- Fold the arms at the elbows and place your left elbow under your right one. Then twist the left arm around the right arm. Try to place the palms together so that they resemble the beak of an eagle, or Garuda. Gaze at a fixed point in front of you so that you can balance better.

III- Slowly bend the leg and lower the body as far as you are able, while keeping balance. Maintain this final pose for a short time and then slowly return to the starting position.

IV- Repeat with the right arm wrapped around the left arm and the left leg wrapped around the right leg.

Anjaneyăsana

CRESCENT MOON POSE' is very good for your legs, strengthening the upper and lower thigh muscles. The asana opens your hips and stretches your front; your back, neck and shoulders. . You will notice, doing it with the knee above the floor and bringing the pelvis down, you need to bring some work into balancing yourself.

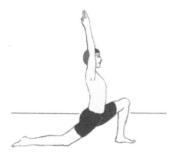

I - Stand straight. Bend forward and place both hands onto the floor beside your feet.

II - Bring your right foot backwards. Optionally you can keep your knee off the floor but bring your pelvis as much down towards the floor as possible. Keep your left knee above the left heel.

III - Bring your hands straight up and stretch them above your head. Bend your back backwards and look up. Breathe normally. This is the final pose.

IV - To come out of the posture, bring your arms down, put your hands on the floor and slowly come up again.

V - Perform the exercise from the other side, too.

Sirsăsana

HEADSTAND POSE' makes the blood flow more easily to the upper parts of the body and the head which are now down, supplying purifying and cleansing fresh oxygen. You will realize that you can concentrate better and your memory improves. Your ears, eyes and nose benefit from the circulation as well. As a result the face becomes radiant and relaxed and the eyes sparkle. Stagnant blood in the legs, and in the pelvic; and abdominal organs is drained of blood and so can be freshly replaced. Sirsăsana provides relief in ocular disorders, premature greying of hair, blood- and menstrual disorders, and the like. There is hardly any ailment which cannot be cured by its performance, but patients of heart disease and high blood pressure are strictly forbidden the practice until some other yogic techniques have cured these diseases.

Beginners can practice near a wall by placing the back of the head a little more than thirty centimeters from the wall in the starting position.

The wall is to be used only to prevent any backward overbalance and not to perform the ăsana. When you gain confidence discard the wall and practice in the middle of an open uncluttered space. Aim to stay in the final position for at least three minutes, since it takes a minute or so for the inverted position to bring changes in the body. Do not stay for more than a maximum of five minutes.

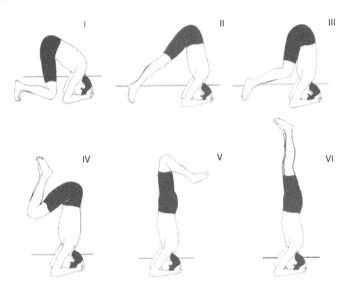

I - Kneel on the ground with the feet a little apart. Interlock your fingers and place the forearms flat on the floor forming a triangle. Place your head halfway between forehead and crown in front of the clasped hands. Wrap the interlocked hands around the back of the head and adjust them to firmly support the head acting as a framework.

II - Straighten your legs and slowly walk the toes to the head as far as possible. Adjust yourself so that you feel comfortable then proceed to raise the feet.

III - Slowly bend the legs keeping the trunk vertical. Bring your thighs as close as possible to the chest. Raise one foot, then the second about twenty centimeters.

IV - Slowly raise your legs further upwards, folding the legs so the heels move towards the buttocks.

V - Raise the knees upwards while keeping the heels near the buttocks, with the feet pointing downwards.

VI - Raise the feet up and straightening the legs. Keep the whole body vertical and make sure that you feel perfect balance. Most of the weight is supported on the head while the arms are used to maintain balance. Relax the whole body and don't point the toes upwards. Close the eyes and breathe deep and slow. With practice you will become as stable as in the standing position.

VII - Return to the starting position on the floor in the reverse order. The body should be lowered slowly and with control, so gently that the feet make no sound when they touch the floor.

VIII - Then sit in a kneeling position with your head on the ground and the arms next to the buttocks (Child Pose) for about thirty seconds.

Utthanpadăsana

THE RAISED LEG POSE' strengthens the abdominal muscles, the digestive system and your lower back.

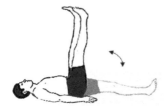

I - Inhale and raise your right leg as high as you can have it go, while keeping it straight with a relaxed foot. Hold it there for a few moments, making sure the other leg remains straight and in touch with the floor. Exhale and slowly lower the leg.

II - Repeat this movement five times and then raise the other leg in the same way for five repetitions.

III - Then hold your hands with the palms down under the buttocks (to give support to your lower back), and slowly raise both legs together repeatedly until you have completed the five rounds with both your legs moving simultaneously

Sarvāngāsana

SHOULDER STAND.' Sarvāngāsana literally means a 'pose for all the parts of the body.' It is one of the many inverted poses of yoga, all of which are extremely beneficial. These inverted āsanas work by reversing the effects of gravity on certain parts of the body, and this pose works its benefits on most.

Due to gravity our lower lungs get most of the oxygen when we breathe. Only when we take a deep breath do our upper lungs also get to play their part. Inverted āsanas also direct oxygen to the upper lung, ensuring healthier lung tissue.

The Sarvāngāsana exercise allows the blood vessels of the feet to return the blood effortlessly to the heart, helps to prevent and reduce varicose veins (veins that have become enlarged and twisted) by reducing the pressure on the legs, and also improves circulation of blood in general. As a result, a large number of dermatological disorders are cured. Sarvāngāsana also pushes healthy, oxygen-rich blood directly into the neck, strengthening the thyroid glands. And, under normal circumstances the heart has to work hard to ensure blood gets pushed upward into the head, but during Sarvāngāsana the heart gets relief as the blood is directly sent to the brain without so much of effort. Patients of high blood pressure are warned against its practice till their blood pressure has been normalized by other yogic practices.

The practice of Sarvāngāsana makes the spine resilient. It builds strength and structure in your back, making it straighter, and tension in your neck, shoulders and the lower back is relieved. This in turn bestows health, beauty, and rejuvenation to the body. Hence, in the discipline of Yoga, particular attention is paid to keep the spine healthy and resilient.

The practice of this asana makes the waist slim, and is the foremost amongst the āsanas for reducing obesity. The paunch vanishes, the body becomes beautiful, the eyes radiant, and the face relaxed. It can be usefully practiced by all; children, young and old persons, and the likes; only patients of heart diseases or of high blood pressure must perform it under the surveillance of an accomplished teacher.

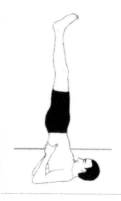

I - Lie flat on your back with your legs straight and together. Straighten your arms and place them beside the body with the palms facing downwards.

II - Raise your legs and buttocks using the abdominal muscles and pressing the hands and arms against the floor. If you find difficulty in raising the legs while keeping them straight, bend the legs, lift your buttocks and bring your knees above your face. Support your back with the hands and only then straighten your legs straight up, fold your forearms upwards, placing your hands on the back and side of the chest. Gently push the chest forwards so that it presses against the chin.

III - Lift your body as high up as possible; making sure that it is resting on your shoulders and not on your back. Your elbows may tend to move outwards and if they do, bring them in.

IV - Straighten your legs and align your hips, feet and shoulders. If this requires muscular effort, slightly incline the legs over the top of the head.

V - The body is supported by the shoulders, neck and back of the head while the arms provide stability. Breathe deep and slow. Do not move your head or turn it to either side and stay in this final pose for as long as is comfortable only.

VI - To come out of the pose, fold your straight legs behind the back of the head, release your hands, place the arms flat on the floor and lower your buttocks while you rotate the legs over the top of the head lowering them to the floor.

Retain the breath either inside or outside while raising and lowering the body, the movement controlled and graceful. Practise a counter pose (for example bhujangăsana, chakrăsana or matsyăsana) for a minute in order to remove the tension in the neck.

Halăsana

PLOUGH POSE' is both a forward bending and a semi-inverted pose. As other inverted postures, it enhances the blood flow to the head. The plough pose makes the entire spine supple; it stretches the spinal column, shoulder muscles and hamstrings. That is why it is beneficial against back pain and helps against stress and fatigue as well as insomnia and head ache caused by tension in those muscles. The nerves both inside and outside the spinal column are strengthened, which leads to better efficiency of all the organs in the body.

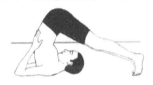

I - Lie on your back with the legs straight and together, the arms on the sides of your body.

II - Raise the two legs to the vertical position using the abdominal muscles. The final pose of Sarvăngăsana can also be used as the starting position for Halăsana.

III - Then fold the legs over the top of the head keeping them straight. Gently lower the feet toward the ground behind the head, touching your toes to the ground.

IV - The hands and arms can be either flat on the floor behind and to the side of the back, or the arms folded behind the back of the head with the hands clasped together, or the hands placed behind the hips. Relax the whole body, keeping the legs straight. Breathe slowly and deeply. This is the final pose.

V - Return to the starting position by first placing the arms flat on the floor behind the back, then performing the steps in reverse.

There are many variations of Halăsana, all of which have distinctive benefits. These variations can be practised individually or one after the other, all performed from the final pose of the Halăsana.

I - Lower Back Stretch: Move the toes gradually nearer towards the back of the head. The legs should be kept straight and together. Grasp the toes with the hands.

II - Upper Back And Neck Stretch: Gradually push the toes as far away from the head as is comfortably possible. Placed the hands behind the hips. Keep the legs straight and together. In the final pose there will be a tight chin lock.

III - Anchored Backstretch: place the arms on the floor behind the head. Grasp the big toes with the fingers. Gradually push the toes as far away from the head as is comfortably possible.

IV - Neck Stretch: this variation is widely known as pasinee mudra (folded mudra). Separate your legs about half a meter. Bend your legs and bring the knees as close as possible to your shoulders with the knees on the ground and the top of your feet flat on the ground. Wrap your arms around the back of your knees and the head. This is the final pose.

V - Neck Tensing Pose. Place both arms behind your back on the floor. Interlock the fingers and push the feet away as far as is comfortable. Press the arms and hands against the floor slightly raising the neck, supporting your weight on the back of your head, shoulders, the arms and the hands.

VI - Pelvic Stretch: hold the big toes with the fingers of each hand. Keeping the legs straight and spread the legs on either side of the head, the toes touching the floor. Separate the legs as much as possible without straining. This is the final pose.

Halăsana and any of the variations can be practised for up to five minutes. We suggest the following sequence: Sarvăngăsana, Halăsana, some or all of the variations followed by any backward bending ăsanas as a counter pose, for example Matsyăsana.

Matsyăsana

FISH POSE.' If you use a little imagination you can see that the folded legs in Matsyăsana resemble the tail of a fish. A special feature is that in this posture it is possible to rest in water without drowning. The folded legs move the centre of gravity nearer the head, allowing it to be held higher above the water and the body becomes more compact and rigid because of the folded legs, enabling to float with much less effort.

Matsyăsana stretches your neck and back muscles in a way that you don't normally do in your daily chores. The spine becomes resilient. It massages the abdominal organs relieving constipation. The ribcage is stretched allowing the chest to expand fully. This asana is also effective for ailments of the throat like tonsillar diseases, and by bending back your head, you stimulate and activate the 'Vishuddhi Chakra' or 'Throat Chakra.' Matsyăsana is an excellent counter pose for forward bending ăsanas and the ideal counter pose for Sarvăngăsana.

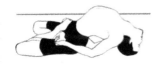

I - Sit in Padmăsana. (see chapter on 'meditation') Lean slightly backwards and place the hands on the floor a little behind and to the side of the buttocks.

II - Bend one of the arms, resting the forearm and elbow on the floor; to do this you will have to twist your body to one side. Then bend the other arm resting both elbows on the floor.

III - Bend your head backwards so that you can see the floor behind your head. Slide your arms forwards and lower the top of the head on the floor. Gently allow the top of the head to support the body weight. Adjust the position of the head to attain the maximum arch of the back.

IV - Then relax the arms, allowing the head, the buttocks and legs to support the weight of the body. Try to grasp the big toes with the hands; if this is too difficult place the hands on the thighs or on the floor. Close your eyes. Breathe deep and slow. This is the final pose.

V - Return to the starting position by using the arms to raise the body back to the upright position.

The following two variations are simplified forms that can be done by those who can't sit in Padmǎsana.

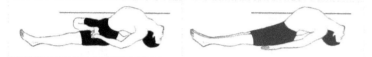

I - Sit on the floor and fold one of the legs into Ardha Padmǎsana (half lotus pose) keeping the other leg straight.

II - Lie on the floor with both legs straight and your arms at the sides of the body with the palms facing down. Put your palms under your buttocks, then lift up your chest and look at your toes. Bend your head backwards and look at the floor behind the head. Gently lower the head to the floor, holding your weight on the arms and the head only touching.

Chakrǎsana

WHEEL POSE.' It is claimed that old age is delayed by the practice of the 'Chakrǎsana. Premature stiffening of the spine is countered by this ǎsana, which is therefore highly important. It directly affects the vertebral column, allowing the body to become resilient and supple, the waist slim, and the chest broad. Chakrǎsana stretches the whole body in a way that it is not stretched normally, which aids the digestive system and bowel movement. Your back also benefits from the turn in the other direction and tension caused by making a hunchback or sitting in one position for a long time is reduced. The backward bend realigns any spinal discs and vertebrae that may be slightly displaced. The asana is especially useful for removing the rigidity of the bones and joints of the ribcage. And this pose strengthens your arms, the knees and the shoulders as they all need to hold your weight!

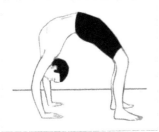

I - Lie on your back. Bend your knees and bring your feet close to your buttocks, placing their soles on the floor in a hip-wide distance of each other.

II - Lift your arms, bend your elbows and place your palms on the floor behind your head, your fingertips pointing towards your legs.

III - With inhalation, you now lift first your buttocks with the strength of the legs and then your torso with the power of your arms and shoulders.

IV - At this point you will feel the blood flowing fast to your head. Straighten your knees and elbows and bring your pelvic area as much towards your hands as you can with the strength or your legs, arching the back as much as possible. Breathe deep and slow. This is the final pose.

V - Return to the starting position by slowly lowering the body to the ground.

Pavana Muktasana

WIND RELEASE POSE.' Wind in the abdomen and indigestion are symptomatic of a poorly functioning gastro-intestinal system. This weakness is relieved by the practice of this asana. Due to the pressure exerted on the abdomen by this asana, the colonic accumulations of gases are pressed out. The posture strengthens the lower back and loosens the vertebrae, and is well suited as a counter pose after exercises that bend your back backward. This posture is not recommended for a person who suffers from high blood pressure, backache or any heart related problems.

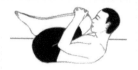

I - Lie on the back with the legs extended. Bend the right knee to the chest and grasp below your knee with fingers interlocked. Keep the other leg straight and in touch with the floor. First, exercise your right leg, thus helping the natural peristalsis of your digestive tract that moves up from the right side, and moves down on the left.

II - Inhale deeply and while holding your breath lift your head and shoulders, touching your right knee with the nose. Remain thus for a few moments before returning your head to the ground while you exhale. Repeat three times and then grasp the other leg.

III - Then, bend both knees bringing the thighs to the chest with the fingers interlocked just below your knees. Raise to touch your nose to the knees for another consecutive three times.

IV - Afterwards relax the whole body in Savăsana with awareness on breath.

Alternatively, you can change your breathing pattern. Exhale deeply before raising the head and hold the breath out while moving into- and remaining in the upward position for a few moments. You breathe in while you move back down.

Naukasana

BOAT POSE.' This is a very good asana for relaxing the muscles and joints of the body. It brings immediate relief to people suffering from nervousness and tension.

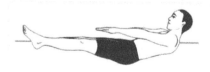

I - Lie flat on the ground facing upwards. Rest your straight arms on the floor beside your body with palms facing downwards.

II - Breathe in deeply and retain the breath inside. Simultaneously raise your legs, arms and shoulders off the ground. Ensure that the arms and legs remain straight. Point your arms towards your feet. Try not to raise the feet or shoulders more than 15 cms from the ground.

III - Stretch and tense the whole body. Feel that every muscle is tensed. Don't strain, but try to hold this raised position for as long as possible, while retaining your breath. Aim at eventually maintaining the raised position for at least a slow count of 10, though at first a count of 2 or 3 is sufficient..

IV - Then allow yourself to slump back to the floor, but without letting your head strike the ground. Let the body sink into the floor. Slowly count from 1 to 60.

This completes 1 round. Perform 3 rounds. After completing 3 rounds of Naukasana remain in the supine pose and relax in Shavasana.

Gomukhǎsana

COW'S FACE POSE.' This practice gives strength to the feet, knees, and waist. The arms and shoulders develop. The chief and unique characteristic of this asana is that it is helpful in diseases of the lungs, because the respiratory movement of the lung on the side on which it is performed is almost stopped and the other lung works more rapidly and vigorously. By alternating its practice, the resting lung can be forced into a state of increased activity. This way the cleansing as well as the blood-circulatory actions on the lungs are started and enhanced. It is possible to inhale markedly greater amounts of oxygen than is ordinarily needed. In this manner, innumerable pores and alveoli of the lungs get cleaned up. It is on this account that yogis have held this asana to be of great usefulness for all types of other practices and for general health improvement.

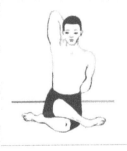

V - Sit on the ground with your left leg bent so that the heel touches your anus. Bend the right leg over the left knee so that the right heel touches the left hip. Take care that your left foot remains straight, touching the ground, and the toes of the right foot also touch the ground. Then raise your right arm, reaching your hand behind the shoulders towards the back. The left arm should be bent upwards behind the back, the hand reaching up, so that the hands meet and all the eight fingers of both the hands are interlocked. In the beginning you may want to use a rope to pull the hands towards each other

VI- Then lower the right elbow as far as possible. During all this, the eyes have to be kept open and the respiration has to go on as usual.

VII- Slowly release your hands and bring your legs back to a straight position before repeating the process by starting on the right side instead.

Makarăsana

CROCODILE POSE' generates subtle energies inside the body and renders it firm and strong like that of a crocodile. Long practice slows down respiration, an achievement of great importance to the yogis. Although resembling a ferocious animal (the crocodile), it is in reality associated with wonderful and miraculous attributes. The asana generates a submissive, humble, and reverential attitude, perhaps on account of the fact that the process of prostration, used as a greeting amongst the yogis and saints, is similar to this asana. People with irregular and crooked bodies ought to practice it. This position encourages the spine to resume its normal shape and releases compression of the spinal nerves. There are a few variations in which this relaxation pose can be performed but it is essential that the abdomen, chest and thighs continue touching the ground fully in any of the following 3 variations.

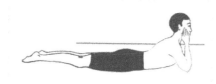

I- Lie flat on the stomach with the hands under the head on top of each other with the palms facing down and one cheek touching the

back of your hand; elbows pointing to the sides; heals apart and big toes touching each other. Breathe normally, close the eyes and relax.

II - Lie flat on the stomach with the head and shoulders raised; heals apart and big toes touching each other; the head is cupped in the palms with the elbows resting on the floor. Breathe normally, close the eyes and relax.

III - Lie flat on the stomach with the arms crossed, your right hand on the left shoulder, left hand on the right shoulder and your head and face tilted to one side. Heals apart and big toes touching each other. Breathe normally, close the eyes and relax.

Pascimottănăsana

BACK STRETCHING POSE' harmonizes pranic energies within the body and the practice of this pose ensures proper circulation of blood in the whole body. The spine becomes resilient, which in turn cures many diseases, relieving arthritis, sciatica, and backache, pain in the knees, the thighs and the legs. It loosens the hip joints and the waist becomes supple. It strengthens and stretches your leg muscles and hamstrings leading to more flexibility. You can feel its work in the muscles and nerves from your toes to your neck. Those who have heavy thighs and buttocks can derive extraordinary benefit from its practice. Dermatological (skin) diseases are cured and the odours of the body are removed and a pleasant aroma is generated. The face becomes radiant and the mind gets repose. Irritable persons are advised to practice this asana. It also induces a keen appetite for food. Further, a variety of worms infesting the gut get killed and eradicated.

The usefulness of this asana is in direct proportion to the length of time it is practised. It is one of those ăsanas which could be practised for hours together! This asana should not be performed with jerks, or after meals.

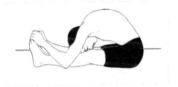

I - Sit on the floor with your legs stretched out in front of the body. Place your hands on the floor with the palms facing down. Hold your back and neck straight.

II - Breathe in deeply and lift your hands from the sides straight up. Then, while exhaling, bend forwards. Grab your big toes with the fingers or feet, and try to touch your forehead to the knees. If you cannot reach your toes, grab your legs wherever you can reach them and bend forward as much as is possible for you

III - Stay in this position. Keep your legs straight and consciously relax your back muscles. As you breathe out, gently pull your back a little further forwards paying attention to only use your arms, keeping the back muscles passive.

IV - Then breathe in while slowly returning to the starting position.

Purvottanăsana

INCLINED PLANE POSE.' Besides improving body balance the 'Purvottanăsana stretches and strengthens your spine, your lower back, upper back, arms, shoulders, thighs and your calf muscles. The weight of the body is held by the wrists and ankles and so they become stronger through the practice of this pose

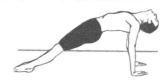

I - Sit on the floor, legs stretched in front of you, the feet a little apart. Arms behind your back a little behind the shoulders with the fingers towards the front or sides. Lean back until you can support your weight on your hands. Do not bend the arms.

II - Exhale, retain the breath and then gradually rise from the ground supporting your weight on your palms and heels.

III - Inhale and push your pelvis up as much as you can. Bend your head towards the back and look behind you. Place the toes on the ground. The sole will then tend to be on the ground on its whole length

Ustrăsana

CAMEL POSE.' According to the teaching of yoga, good health, longevity, and the absence of disease are in direct proportion to the suppleness and resilience of the spine and the Ustrăsana has definite advantages for the vertebral column. It is given a backward bend, loosening up the vertebrae and helping to correct rounded shoulders and a stooping back. Backache, neck ache or general stiffness in the spine will be relieved through regular practice of Ustrăsana. The spine becomes resilient.

The shoulders and the neck are strengthened while making the waist slim. It is a panacea for persons with paunches and heavy buttocks. The practice of this asana stimulates the abdominal organs and can relieve constipation and help those who suffer from flatulence.

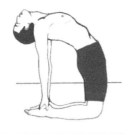

I - Kneel on your heels and separate the knees and feet so that they are a shoulder-width apart from each other

II - Lean slightly back, turn to the right side and grasp the right heel with the right hand and straighten your arm. Then square your body and grasp the other heel with the left hand.

III - Press your heels down with the hands, push your pelvis to the front to increase the arch, your chest upwards and let your head hang back.

IV - Remain in the final pose for as long as is comfortable. Return by raising your head up, bringing your pelvis back, your chest back, then leave the grip of your heels and slowly sit back down on your heels.

Suptravajrăsana

SUPINE ANKLE POSE' makes the waist resilient and the chest broad. It stretches the pelvic region and will reduce stiffness and rigidity in thighs and legs. It relieves painful conditions of the back and the knees, strengthens the abdominal organs and increases the blood flow to the thighs and buttocks. By improving circulation of blood, it makes for a healthy body. The dormant forces at the base of the spine become active and by regular practice your relaxation deepens. This asana relieves fatigue.

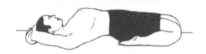

I - Sit straight with your legs stretched and the heels together, and the palms of your hands pressing on the floor by the side of the buttocks.

II - Fold the right leg at the knee and place the heel under the right buttock. Then the left leg. Keep your knees together and rest the palms on the upper thighs.

III - Slowly recline backwards and rest your right elbow on the ground, keeping the entire body weight on the right elbow first, and then as you recline further, on both elbows.

IV - Exhale and lie on your back resting your arms and hands along the side of the body. Keep the knees close together touching the ground. Breathe normal and stay in this final pose for some time. You can also cross your hands under your head, using them as a pillow.

V - To come out of the pose, breathe in and return to the support on your elbows, slowly come back to Vajrăsana (position II), and unfold the legs one by one.

Bhujangăsana

COBRA POSE' emulates the action of the cobra raising itself just prior to striking at its prey. Practicing the cobra pose is very good for strengthening the spinal column and the muscles supporting the spine. This is how it is often recommended against backache, but patients of hernia are strictly warned against its practice. The pose also works wonders for your abdomen and abdominal organs. It helps your digestion and relieves constipation, indigestion, and flatulence. The practice of the Bhujangăsana makes the waist slender and the chest broad, helping the lungs to fully expand and collect a larger amount of oxygen which then helps the heart and blood circulation. The result is that you feel fitter, more energetic and the body becomes beautiful. This is equally useful to all men, women, and children; young and old; the healthy or the sick.

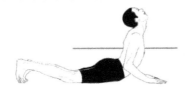

I - Lie flat on the stomach with the legs straight. Place the hands with the palms on the floor at the side of the shoulders with the fingers pointing forwards and the arms bent with the elbows pointing back. Your toes should point to the back, so that the soles of your feet are turned upwards. Rest the forehead on the ground, close your eyes and relax the whole body.

II - Breathe in and raise the body by straightening the arms until even the navel does not touch the floor anymore. Bend your head backwards and look straight up.

III - Your arms may or may not be straight—it depends on the flexibility of your back. Your legs and feet should remain together and touching each other. Keep your shoulders relaxed. This is the final pose. Do complete yogic breathing while you are in the pose.

IV - Hold for as long as comfortable and return to the starting position on an exhalation.

Shalabhăsana

LOCUST POSE.' Just as the locusts have a distinctive and highly developed faculty of hopping high, the practice of this asana perfects many of man's faculties. Shalabhăsana is an excellent backward bending ăsana for improving the health and strength of the lower back and has a specific influence on the organs, muscles and nerves of the pelvis, abdomen and chest. The chest broadens and the heart is directly massaged. The waist becomes resilient and supple. It is also very useful for the shoulders and abdomen, relieving constipation and stimulating digestion. The practice of the locust posture affects the fine tissues and haemo circulatory channels instead of affecting the gross masses of muscles as most other exercises do. The navel assumes its normal position; the asana helps in the development and expression of Manipura Chakra or Navel Chakra.

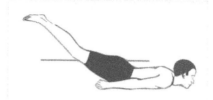

I- Lie on your abdomen with your chin on the ground with your legs straight and the feet together. Hold your arms beside the body with the hands under your pelvis and the palms facing downwards, upwards or clenched.

II- Inhale deeply, hold your breath and raise the legs straight up, keeping them together without bending your knee or your ankles by the use of pressure on the arms and contracting the lower back muscles.

III- Hold your breath and keep your legs in the raised position for as long as you can without any strain.

IV- Then slowly lower your legs and exhale, relax for a few moments and then repeat the practice for a second time.

Easier than Shalabhăsana is the ARDHA SHALABHĂSANA (ardha ~half), Half Locust Pose,. The technique is the same, except that first one leg is raised in step II through IV and then the other, repeating the sequence for each leg.

Dhanurăsana

BOW POSTURE.' Practice of this asana removes constipation and stimulates the gastric secretions. It also relieves ache or colic of the abdomen. A distinctive and important aspect of this asana is that it restores the displaced `navel' to its normal position. It stretches the entire front body from the ankles to the throat and if the abdomen or buttocks have become corpulent, it must be practiced for 10 to 15 minutes daily.

The spine becomes resilient. It is useful as a general preventive against disease if practiced daily, but patients of hernia should avoid it.

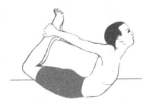

I - Lie on your abdomen, then bend your legs and grasp the ankles. Let the toes touching each other and place your chin on the ground.

II - Inhale and arch your back by lifting your thighs, chest and head off the ground using the leg muscles. Keep your arms straight, the abdomen in contact with the floor and breathe normally. Stay for as long as is comfortable.

III - Relax the leg muscles and return to the starting position. When you reach the ground, breathe out and relax.

Balăsana

CHILD POSE.' In this asana the body faces the floor in a fetal position. The knees and hips are bent with the shins on the floor. The chest can rest either on the knees or the knees can be spread to allow the chest to go between the knees. The head is stretched forward towards the ground - the forehead may touch the ground. The arms may be stretched forward in front of the head or backwards towards the feet.

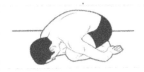

I - Kneel on the floor. Touch your big toes together and sit on your heels, then separate your knees about as wide as your hips.

II - Exhale and lay your torso down between your thighs.

III - Lay your hands on the floor alongside your torso, palms up, and release the fronts of your shoulders toward the floor. Feel how the weight of the front shoulders pulls the shoulder blades wide across your back.

Meru Vakrăsana

SPINAL TWIST.' In India the spine is known as the merudand, which means 'mountainous stick', for the vertebrae of the spine jut out like a range of mountains. This Meru Vakrăsana twists the whole spine from top to bottom, loosening up all the vertebrae, and strengthens and firms the nerves within and surrounding the spine.

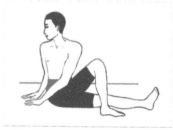

I - Sit straight with your legs stretched. Bend your left leg and place your foot on the outside of the right knee with the sole flat on the floor.

II - Place the right palm behind your back on the floor with the fingers pointing back, twist the upper body to the right and grasp the right ankle with the left hand holding your arm straight and touching the outside of the right knee and calf.

III - Turn your head to the right and look over your shoulder. Push your upper body straight with your right arm, align your shoulders and breathe normally.

IV - Inhale deeply and with exhalation slowly twist the trunk further to the right by levering the left arm against the right leg;

V - Stay in the final pose for a little while, then return to the starting position and repeat the same with your other side.

Ardha Matsyendrăsana

HALF SPINAL TWIST.' This ăsana is named after the great yogi Matsyendranath. The `serpent power' or the 'Kundalini Sakti,' which is instrumental in enabling the yogis to scale the ultimate heights of yoga, is speedily `awakened' through the practice of this posture. Until your back becomes more flexible, practice the simpler ăsana Meru Vakrăsana.

The Matsyendrăsana stimulates gastric secretion. It is an efficient instrument for combating serious ailments. Flatulence, chronic enlargement of the spleen as well as disorders of the liver are relieved by this asana. It is most beneficial for intestinal disorders. Matsyendrăsana is also the only yogic asana which cures helminthiasis, the disease produced by the infestation of the body, specially the gastrointestinal tract, by worms of various types which are usually difficult to get rid of. The continuous practice of Matsyendrăsana results in extermination of these infections, by killing the worms as well as by causing them to be expelled. This ăsana also applies torsion to the upper body, useful for reducing the tendency of adjoining vertebrae to fuse together.

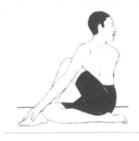

I- Sit on the floor with both legs straight. Bend your right knee and place the sole of your foot flat on the floor on the outside of the left knee. Then bend your left knee to your right and place your foot next to your right hip.

II- Exhale and twist your upper body to the right, bringing your left shoulder past of the right knee and place your left hand on the right foot grabbing your toes.

III- Place the right palm behind your back on the floor with the fingers pointing back, push your upper body vertical and turn your head. Look over and above your right shoulder keeping your shoulders in line. Breathe normally.

IV- Stay in the final position for some time, then return to the starting position and straighten both legs. Repeat the twisting of the body to the other side.

If you find Ardha Matsyendrăsana easy to do, then you can do a more difficult form: Instead of grasping your right ankle with your left hand, push your left hand and arm underneath the bent right leg through the space between the calf and thigh. A little bit of adjustment may be necessary, but it is possible to reach backwards behind the back with the left hand and then to fold your right arm behind the back and grasp the hands behind the back.

Kakăsana

CROW POSE.' Develops the faculty of keeping the body in balance and is held by the Yogis to be an important means of inducing mental concentration. The arms, shoulders and hands acquire great strength through the practice of this asana. If you practice Kakăsana regularly, you will less likely have tension and pain in your upper back, neck and shoulders. Ailments of the shoulders are cured and it builds up cardiac reserves as well.

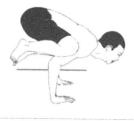

I - Squat down with your feet a few inches apart from each other. If you can, touch your buttocks with your heels. Open your knees hip-wide apart and place your hands in front of your feet with the elbows in between your knees.

II - In the next step you bend your elbows and place your knees on your upper arm. Now slowly shift your body weight onto your arms, lift your heels and with exhalation come forward and on your toes. Bit by bit you shift your weight further and lift your toes from the floor.

III - Point your toes back, look to the front and smile. This is the final pose. Stay in the final pose for a comfortable length of time.

There are many variations to this balancing pose, all carrying the same name. One alternative to the basic form of Kakăsana is the 'High Crow';

I - Take the starting position as in step I of the basic crow.

II - Then, instead of leaning forward, come up on your toes and place your knees as high as possible on your upper arm, in your armpit.

III - Lean forward and lift your feet off the ground finding your balance. Then point your feet up and straighten your elbows. Look at the floor or slightly forward and breathe normally.

Mayurăsana

PEACOCK POSE' removes all maladies of the abdomen. A peacock has the ability to absorb and destroy toxins in the things that it eats. This pose is renowned for its capacity to eliminate toxins from the body. It helps in reducing to ashes the excessive and unwholesome quantities of food, and, by stimulating and generating the digestive 'fire' of the stomach, even the bitterly poisonous elements are annihilated. The peacock feasts on a venomous creature like the serpent without being afflicted by its poison, and not only digests it but also prefers it to all other food. It is believed that the peacock eats more than any other bird and that the 'fire' of its stomach remains ablaze all the time. Constipation and flatulence can be cured in faithful practice. It is equally effective against chronic enlargements and other disorders of the spleen as well as for diseases of the liver and indigestion. It is claimed in the classics on yoga that with its help even poison can be easily assimilated and a person who can practice it for 1520 minutes at a stretch becomes immune to the poisonous effects of snakes and scorpions just as the peacock is.

The peacock pose is a balancing ăsana that will make your arms and hands extremely strong and it is highly beneficial for the lungs as well. It is however very easy to fall forward from the final pose, so if necessary place a small cushion under your face on the floor.

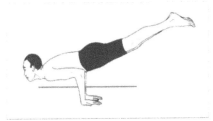

I - Kneel on the floor with the two feet together and separate the knees. Place both your palms on the floor between the knees with the fingers pointing back with the wrists and forearms touching each other.

II - Lean forward and rest your abdomen on the top of the elbows just below the navel and your chest on top of the upper arms. Stretch your legs back straight and together.

III - Inhale and tense the muscles of the body, elevate your upper body, head and legs so that they lie in one straight, horizontal line. Hold your head up and balance on the palms using the fingers for corrections. This is the final pose.

IV - Hold the final pose for as long as is comfortable. Then slowly lower the legs to the ground and return to the starting pose.

A variation of Mayurāsana which can be done by those who can sit in Padmāsana is called PADMA MAYURĀSANA (Padma ~lotus). 'Lotus or Bound peacock pose'.

I - Sit in Padmāsana. Raise the body onto the knees. Place the palms flat on the floor in front of the body; fingers pointing backwards

II - Bend the elbows and bring them together; lean forwards and place them against each side of the abdomen; lean further forwards resting the chest rests on the upper arms

III - Find the balance point of the body; lean further forwards and raise the folded legs; make the trunk, head and legs lie in one horizontal straight line; either hold your breath or breathe slowly and deeply. This is the final pose. Stay for a comfortable time.

Titli Āsana

BUTTERFLY POSE' is so called because the legs move up and down like a butterfly's wings. It is good for the spine and lower back as well as your hip joints. The pose loosens the rigidity of the muscles and tendons in the groins and strengthens the muscles of your hips and legs and makes your hamstrings more flexible. It is a good asana in preparation for the meditational pose Padmasana.

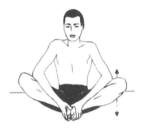

I- Sit on the floor with your legs extended in front of the body. Bend the legs sideways and place the soles of both feet together.

II- Hold your feet with the hands and place your elbows inside the tops of the thighs.

III- Gently push the knees of both legs towards the ground, using your elbows as levers; push the knees as close as possible to the floor. After a short duration release the legs. Repeat for about 10 to 20 times.

IV- Release the hands but keep the legs and feet in the same position. Place your hands on the knees and push the knees up and down using your arms. Repeat for about 20 to 40 times.

Kriyas, Mudras and Bandhas

KRIYA yoga is a system of purifying the whole mind-body. On our way to physical well-being, it is important we part with any impurities that have been allowed to enter our system. Without a purified body, one will not be ready for the higher practices of yoga.

Mudras are special physical positions of the body or parts of the body. They are a combination of subtle physical movements that alter mood, attitude and perception, deepening awareness and concentration.

Bandhas are a small but essential part of yoga, where they are combined with various other yogic techniques. Traditional yogic texts speak of psychic blocks and mental problems that prevent an individual entering into meditation. These blocks or knots have to be removed if one wants to know the experience of higher awareness. Bandhas are particularly effective in breaking open or removing these blocks.

Kriyas

IN the Science of Yoga as much importance is given to certain yogic cleansing processes called 'kriyăs' as is to ăsanas or prănăyăma. This chapter is devoted to a description of these cleansing methods. If there is excessive impurity in your body then there will be a drastic purging process and if you suffer from any serious physical illness, then we strongly suggest that you do not attempt Kriya yoga, for it may easily worsen the condition. Take steps to cure your illness by adopting any suitable healing systems, possibly Hatha Yoga.

The yogic kriyăs evolved in times before cleaner sanitary conditions, refrigeration, and clean food were commonplace as they are today in many countries. Although they may have been more necessary back then, the kriyăs remain useful and valuable techniques today. They are very important for physical and mental health, and these simple techniques will help to overcome internal disorders. Especially if we have not been as good to our bodies as we should have been. Follow a clean and healthful diet, and never use the kriyăs as antidotes to overeating or bad dietary habits.

There are six main groups of Kriyăs or Shat-Kriyăs (literally, the six practices or rites.) They help to become more intimate with our own body's internal processes, and invite wellness and self-healing. The shat-kriyăs are Neti, which is water or string cleansing of the nasal passages; Nauli, the churning or pumping of the stomach; Dhauti, or the cleansing of the stomach, teeth, throat, and rectum; Vasti, or colon cleansing similar to an enema; Trătaka, which is gazing at a candle flame or small object; and Kapalbhati, a breathing technique to cleanse and strengthen the lungs.

Neti

JALA Neti' is a Kriya for cleaning the nasal and sinus cavity by the use of water. Other types of Neti that are in general practice are; 'Dugdha Neti' using milk and 'Ghrta Neti,' using ghee. In our nose there is hair and mucus that catches dust and dirt, preventing the impurities from reaching further into your respiratory system. Neti helps to properly clean your nose from this dust, mucus and bacteria, which may be caught in your nose. Neti not only clears the nasal passages but also improves resistance to many irritants. Other reasons for the use of Neti are the stimulation of nerve endings in the nose which leads to improvement in the brain and organs to which these nerves connect and is particularly effective in cases of forgetfulness. Neti is excellent for cases of chronic headache, insomnia and drowsiness. Diseases specific to the nose are effectively bettered. Affections of the eye such as soreness, night-blindness, and dimness of eyesight, diseases of the ear, impaired hearing and discharge through the ear can all be relieved. In short all the diseases of the different organs from the neck upward can be effectively treated with the help of this exercise.

For doing Neti, you need a jug with one pint capacity with a spout or nozzle from which you can pour out water in a steady stream that can be inserted in the nostrils with ease. It can be made of any material that does not contaminate water.

I - Fill your neti pot with half a liter of pure lukewarm water and mix about one teaspoon of sea salt into the water.

II - Squat on the ground and hold the jug of water in the palm of your hand. Tilt your head and insert the spout in one nostril and bend your head in the direction of the other nostril. Start breathing through your mouth. Relax and let the water flow into one nostril and out of the other. If you breathe through the nostrils, the water you are pouring in will get into the upper regions with considerable discomfort. When the water is all out, repeat the same procedure from the other nostril.

III - After completing these steps, get up and bend forward at an angle of 90 degrees. Breathe in and out sharply through the nose while moving your head right, left, up and down. This will help you eliminate whatever water remains.

IV - Now tilt your head back for about 30 seconds, then to the left for 30 seconds and finally to the right for 30 seconds. Again, you sniff anything out that still remained inside.

Nauli

NAULI (control of the abdominal recti) is an excellent example of developing control over those muscles which we hardly use individually and about whose separate identity the majority of people are not even aware. Nauli is a yogic technique of massaging the entire abdomen and stomach. It is very beneficial for the health of the digestive system, and of all yogic practices, Nauli gives the most profound massage to the inner organs. This is achieved by contracting and rolling the abdominal muscles; the rectus abdominis which form the front linear wall of the abdominal cavity, is used with other muscles like the trans versus abdominis etc. It is quite difficult to acquire, and time and regular practice are required in order to develop control over these muscles and master Nauli, but with determination, it can be done by almost everyone. The exercise of contracting the recti individually and independently really depends on a willful dissociation of their functions from the other adjoining groups of muscles. Through its accomplishment, great control can be acquired on the pressure dynamics of the abdomen. The rotation of the recti results in improving the mobility of the various organs located in the abdominal cavity, and in increasing the circulation. The nerve plexuses and their fine terminals are all activated as welll. Of even greater importance to its accomplishment, is the capacity to produce negative pressure in the abdomen. This on the one hand sucks up more blood in the abdomen and on the other allows greater control on the rates at which various substances can be ejected out of the system. The technique to acquire nauli is divided into stages so as to firstly gain control over the associated muscles, and then to operate them in the required fashion.

Madhyama nauli (central contraction)

I - Stand slightly bent forward with your hands on your knees and legs about a meter apart.

II - After exhaling and emptying the lungs as much as possible, completely draw in your stomach. Pressing down with your arms, draw up the abdominal muscles (uddiyăna bandha) at the same time forcing the rectus abdominis (Nala) to stand out in isolation.

III - Try to contract the muscles as much as possible, but do not strain. Hold the contraction for as long as you are able to comfortably retain the breath. While doing this exercise, look at the abdomen to see how far you have succeeded in your attempt.

IV - Then relax the muscles of the abdomen so that you return to uddiyăna bandha. Breathe in slowly and let the abdomen expand.

Repeated attempts will at last be crowned with success and the rectus abdomini will stand out. Failure at the initial stages should not discourage you.

Vama daksina-nauli

V - When you are successful in getting your rectus abdominis to stand out, you have only to lean on the left and it will move to the left or on the right and it will move in that direction. It will then be easy to revolve it and make it describe a circle.

VI - Once you are able to do this make the rectus abdominis describe three and a half circles to the left, then an equal number to the right. This completes this exercise.

Dhauti

ANY of these techniques called 'Dhauti' will be familiar, while others you may never have considered before. Dhauti are techniques for cleansing the digestive tract up to the stomach. These remove excess and old bile, mucus and toxins, infectious bacteria, and restore the natural balance of the body. Dandă Dhauti consists of a series of simple practices which clean various organs and regions of the head; Jala dhauti (also known as vamana dhauti) is a technique for cleaning the digestive tract, and Vastra Dhauti is a method of cleaning the throat, oesophagus and stomach,

Dandă Dhauti

THESE practices, as well as jala neti, effect directly or indirectly the main senses of the body—hearing, seeing, smelling and tasting. The ancient yogis realized the necessity of maintaining the sensory organs in optimum condition.

I - Danta dhauti—the cleaning of the teeth and gums with a special stick, usually of neem or babool. A soft bristled toothbrush and paste can also be used. Clean your teeth at least twice every day and even better after each meal. Clean the brush as often as possible. Clean the gums with the index finger making a hard, rubbing motion over both the inner and outer gums

II - Jihva dhauti—the cleaning the tongue by rubbing it with the joined first finger and thumb in a downward motion, and then squeezing it. Rub the root of the tongue slowly and thoroughly for a few minutes

III - Karna dhauti—cleaning the ears with the middle finger and nothing smaller,

IV - Kapalrandhra dhauti—cleaning the upper back portion of the palate,

V - Kapal dhauti—Press the temples on each side of the forehead with two thumbs, making small circling movements for a minute or so and then repeat the same movement rotating in the opposite direction.

VI - Chakshu dhauti—bathing the eyes with tepid saline water or urine.

Jala dhauti

JALA dhauti' is a technique for cleaning the digestive tract from the stomach to the mouth by vomiting salty water. In this practice there is no unpleasant taste, smell and nausea as there is during times of sickness.

I - Drink Luke-warm saline water until you can take no more, or feel like vomiting. Stand with the feet together and trunk bent forward at an angle of about 90.

II - Trickle the back of the throat with the middle three fingers to vomit out all the water. Repeat the trickling and vomiting till no more water comes out.

Vastra Dhauti

VASTRA Dhauti' is a method of cleaning the throat, oesophagus and stomach with a length of cloth (Vastra). We recommend learning this practice under the guidance of an instructor.

Vasti

VASTI is a method of cleaninsing the colon by sucking in air (sthala vasti) or water (jala vasti). Traditionally, the yogi would use a thin, hollow bamboo tube inserted into the anus, but is not required. For jala vasti, he would then squat over water to suck in water and perform Madhyama nauli. This produces a vacuum in the abdominal cavity that naturally draws water into the rectum. For air basti no water or bath is required.

If you cannot do vasti (with or without a tube) then use an enema, but you should aim to develop more control over the abdominal muscles in order to practice vasti in the future.

The most common method of using an enema is gravity feed. The liquid used as enema is kept in a container above the level of the anus. A thin tube feeds the water directly into the colon under the force of gravity; no effort is necessary. The gravity feed method is very similar to vasti and is much easier. Basti requires some degree of muscular control.

Trătaka

TO GAZE' is the practice of staring at some external object. This fixed gazing is a method of meditation which involves concentrating on a single point such as a small object, black dot or candle flame. Any object will do, but focus on it and gaze at it without blinking. You can even close your eyes and focus within. It is used in yoga as a way of developing concentration and strengthening the eyes.

As has been said: "When both the life force as well as the mind get absorbed in the Yogi sitting in a state of Trătaka, concentrating his unwavering gaze on the spot illumined like a star, that state is called the superb 'Sambhavi' state." The mastery of the Trătaka technique is called the Sambhavi Mudra.

I - Assuming the Siddhăsana or Padmăsana pose in a dark room, light a candle and place it about 75 to 90 centimeters away from you at the level of your eyes. Focus on the flame and continuously stare at it without blinking until tears start running down your cheeks, and as soon as they do so close your eyes.

II - Then close your eyes but keep gazing at the same point and imagine the same flame from behind your eyelids for 15 to 20 seconds. After that relax your eye muscles.

III - Place your palms over your eyes without any pressure on the eyeballs. Gently move your palms in circles. Take a towel or tissue to wipe your eyes.

IV - Repeat the exercise. When you are able to fix your gaze for 10 or 15 minutes without blinking, you will find that the spot you look as is surrounded by many minor lights. But the gaze must not be deflected from the central spot. When at last you see nothing except light in the direction in which you look, you will have succeeded. Complete mastery will come only when you feel the glow of the light illuminate your own being.

Kapălabhăti

FRONTAL BRAIN CLEANSING' is essentially a system of vigorous respiration and thus combines the advantages of increased oxygen intake as well as aeration and drying of the respiratory passages. It has been demonstrated in some physiological studies into the effects of the various types of respiratory exercise on oxygen consumption, that there are appreciable differences in their results. Kapălabhăti was shown to cause an increase in the oxygen consumption to the extent of 20 percent! The vitalising influence of this technique of breathing is quite evident. The technique invigorates the entire brain and can be used to energize the mind for mental work when you feel tired, and to remove sleepiness. This exercise awakens the dormant centres that are responsible for subtle perception. Kapălabhăti must follow the Jala-neti so as to eliminate whatever water has been left in the nose and is an ideal practice to do immediately before meditation techniques.

I - Sit straight in a comfortable position, close your eyes and breathe rapidly from the abdomen as such: Inhale deeply through your nose. Then push the air out, forcing your abdomen in by contracting your abdominal muscles. By allowing these muscles to release, air flows in automatically without any effort. Focus on the exhalation and repeat a comfortable number of times — no more.

II - Then take one deep and slow breath in and hold your breath for as long as is comfortable.

III - Release your breath and slowly breathe out. Then breathe naturally a few times. This is one round. You can do several rounds as you feel inclined.

Mudras

GESTURES', the translation of 'Mudras,' are special physical positions of the body or parts of the body. They are a combination of subtle physical movements that alter mood, attitude and perception, deepening awareness and concentration. There are many forms of yoga mudras; head mudras, postural mudras, lock mudras and perineal mudras. There are also many hand positions called 'Hasta Mudras' and we will limit our coverage on the subject of mudras to this specific group.

Ancient yogis are often depicted displaying a Hasta Mudra. In yoga, these mudrăs are used in conjunction with prănăyăma or meditation, generally while seated in a meditational pose, to stimulate different parts of the body involved with breathing and to affect the flow of prana. The mudras have symbolic and psychic meaning. If one dwells on the meaning of a mudra, it is possible to invoke inner forces, and if the reader has read the chapter on the subject he will appreciate the significance of prana. Some of this prana is released from the tips of the fingers. The hand mudras are methods of redirecting the prana inwards and the contact with the knees close some pranic circuits keeping the prana within the body. This is why mudras are so powerful and important while meditating. At first it may seem to be an insignificant aspect, yet the wrong position of the hands can restrict successful meditation.

Nasagra Mudra

NOSE MUDRA.' Raising the hands in this position is called 'Nasagra Mudra', the nose tip position, and is used while practicing certain pranayama techniques where the breath through the nostrils is controlled by the fingers of one hand, held in front of the face.

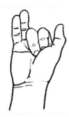

I - Keep your head and back upright without strain and hold your right hand in front of your face, keeping your elbow in front of- and near the chest and the forearm vertical, reducing the tendency of the raised arm to tire. Bend the second (index) and third fingers so that they rest in the palm of the hand.

II - Place the thumb beside the right nostril and the fourth (ring) finger beside the left nostril. The little finger is not used and rests next to the fourth finger.

III - The right nostril can now be left open or closed by pressing the side of the nose with the thumb. This allows air to flow, or prevents the flow. The air flow through the left nostril is controlled with the ring finger.

Chin Mudra and Jnana Mudra

CONSCIOUSNESS AND INTUITIVE KNOWLEDGE MUDRAS.' The symbolic meaning of Chin, 'Consciousness' and Jnana, 'Intuitive Knowledge' Mudras is the same with regard to the meaning of their respective names, and every aspect of these gestures has deep symbolic meaning, but first let us explain how to make these gestures correctly.

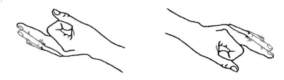

I - Sit in any meditative ăsana. Fold the index fingers. The tips can be placed at the roots- or in contact with the tips of the thumbs. Straighten the small, ring and middle fingers slightly separated.

II - For Chin Mudra, put the backs of the hands on the knees, the palms facing upwards and the three unbent fingers pointing forwards away from the body.

III - In Jnana Mudra, your palms are facing downwards, the unbent fingers and thumbs pointing towards the floor in front of your knees.

The small, ring and middle fingers that are held straight, represent the three categories of nature: tamas (inertia, laziness, darkness, ignorance), rajas (action, passion, movement) and sattwa (understanding, purity). These three states have to be transcended one after the other, in order to pass from darkness into light and from ignorance to knowledge. The bent index finger represents the individual manifestation of consciousness (jivatma). The thumb symbolizes the all pervading consciousness. The individual is bowing down to supreme consciousness acknowledging its unsurpassed power. Yet at the same time the index finger and thumb touch each other, which shows that though they seem separate, in fact the individual being is one with the supreme. It symbolizes yoga at its culmination.

Bandhas

LOCKS.' These exercises are called locks because they make a separation between two parts of the body. Air will not pass from one side of the lock to the other and your energy is rotating in the separated parts, not in between them. The bandhas are considered very important parts of yogic exercise due to their great effect on the body.

The three Bandhas described are; Jalandhara Bandha being the throat lock, Uddiyana Bandha the abdominal lock and Mula Bandha the root lock. When you combine Jalandhara Bandha and Mula Bandha, it is called the Maha Bandha. If you combine all three bandhas together, it is called Maha Mudra. The unity of the three bandhas is called 'Tribandha'

Jalandhara Bandha

THROAT LOCK' is beneficial for the glands in the area of your neck. The bending of your chin will cause the thyroid gland to release a fluid that will increase the number of white blood cells in your blood. This strengthens your immune system. This bandha also increases the strength and the blood flow in your vocal cord, giving you a wonderfully sounding strong voice, good for singers and speakers alike.

1- For practicing this lock, sit in a comfortable position and bend your chin to the collarbone by contracting your throat muscles. The locking will prevent you from bringing outer air in or inner air out. This can be done after inhalation or exhalation.

Mula Bandha

ROOT LOCK', referring to our perineum between the sexual organs and the anus. The perineum is also known as the place where kundalini energy lies in the first chakra, the Mooladhara Chakra. At the perineum is the bottom of our body, the junction and starting place of our nervous system and the three main nadis, ida, pingala and sushumna that carry the kundalini energy up through your body. By performing Mula Bandha, you stimulate both, the nervous system and the energy system, at their roots and beginning. This stimulation brings you a lot of good; it calms your mind, gives you emotional and psychological strength, and makes your mind more stable and balanced.

I- To perform the Mula Bandha, sit in any comfortable position. Contract your perineum towards your navel with inhalation and close your eyes. Focus and visualize the muscles between your pubic bone and coccyx bone, then deepen your breath. You can slowly increase the time holding the contraction.

The contraction is the same feeling as when you need to go to toilet and you are holding the urine in your body. You also use these muscles when you are forcing yourself to urinate even when you don't have to. In the beginning, you can place your finger on those muscles to make sure you are not working with your anal muscle or the muscle of your sexual organ.

Uddiyana Bandha

ABDOMINAL LOCK' is a very beneficial pose for your complete respiratory system. It strengthens your diaphragm and your lungs and helps you to breathe easily after practice. The Apana Vayu, the air located between navel and anus, is regulated which can prevent problems with gas in the intestines. It is also good for Samana Vayu which is the air in the navel region and can cause digestion problems when it is disturbed. Prana Vayu which lies in your heart region will also be regulated and thus acidity and breathing problems are prevented. You see that Uddiyana Bandha is beneficial for your complete upper body.

It increases the digestive fire and detoxifies the digestive tract which improves your whole digestion, helps against colitis and the contraction given by this posture is good for your Solar Plexus and the Manipura Chakra located in this area. When you start practicing this exercise you will quickly notice that it strengthens the abdominal muscles. This bandha can be performed while sitting or standing.

I- Take a deep breath and place your hands on your knees, and while you exhale, lean forward which will help you to press all air out until no air is left in your lungs.

II- After exhalation, hold your breath and contract your abdominal muscles so that your navel is pulled further inside and up, towards your middle back. Stay in that position until you feel like inhaling. For coming out of the pose relax your abdominal muscles and straighten your body while you inhale.

Always exhale from your mouth to get all air out of your body. Do not inhale while trying to keep the posture. When you feel like inhaling, come up and let your lungs fill with air. Take care not to overwork or cross your limits for it could make you dizzy and may even lead to fainting.

Maha Mudra

IN yogic scripture, MAHA MUDRA is said to be one of the greatest postures as it includes all the three bandhas. This gives control and command over your mental and physical constitution. It has all the benefits of the three different locks combined. Before you practice the Maha Mudra, make sure you have practiced the three Bandhas separately and Maha Bandha first. This will ensure you know how they feel, and give your body the opportunity to accustom itself to these locks, and have their individual effects work on your system first.

I - Sit upright with your legs straight. Place your left heel on your perineum. The sole of the left foot touching your right thigh. Take care that your right knee is touching the floor and the leg remains straight throughout. Inhale deeply.

II - Exhale from the mouth, bend forward and make all three bandhas, the Mula Bandha, Uddiyana Bandha and Jalandhara Bandha. This means you contract your perineum muscles, place your chin on your chest and let the vacuum in your abdomen pull your navel up and in.

III - Lean forward to grab your right toes, or if you cannot reach, your ankle or calves with both hands, and hold the air out. Close your eyes and stay in the yoga pose.

IV - For coming out of the pose, release the locks and come up while inhaling. Repeat from the other side.

Pranayama

ALL is in vibration, from the tiniest atom to the greatest sun. In nature, there is nothing in absolute rest. A single atom deprived of vibration would wreck the universe. Matter is being constantly played upon by energy and countless forms and numberless varieties result. Yet, even the forms and varieties are not permanent. They begin to change the moment they are created, and from them are born innumerable new forms, which in turn change and give rise to newer forms, and so on and on, in infinite succession. Nothing is permanent, and the atoms of the human body are also in constant vibration and unceasing changes are occurring. In a few months, there is almost a complete change in the matter composing the body.

In all vibration is to be found a certain rhythm. Rhythm pervades the universe. The swing of the planets around the sun; the rise and fall of the sea; the beating of the heart; the ebb and flow of the tide; all follow rhythmic laws. Our bodies are as much subject to rhythmic laws as is the planet in its revolution around the sun. Much of the Yogi Science of Breath is based upon this known principle of nature. You have heard how a note on a violin, if sounded repeatedly and in rhythm, will start into motion vibrations, which will in time destroy a bridge. The same result is true when a regiment of soldiers crosses a bridge, the order being always given to 'break step' on such an occasion, lest the vibration bring down both bridge and regiment. These manifestations of the effect of rhythmic motion will give you an idea of the effect on the body of rhythmic breathing.

The body which you occupy is like a small inlet running in to the land from the sea. Although apparently subject only to its own laws, it is really subject to the ebb and flow of the tides of the ocean. The great ocean of life is swelling and receding, rising and falling, and we are responding to its vibrations and rhythm. At times the mouth of the inlet seems choked up with debris, we fail to receive the impulse from Mother Ocean, and disharmony manifests within us. By falling in with the rhythm of the body thru prănăyăma, the whole system catches the vibration and becomes in harmony with the will, which causes the rhythmic motion of the lungs. With the body thus attuned in complete harmony, the flow of prana is harmonized and the debris and congestion in the pranic passages (nadis) removed.

Of these nadis, three are particularly important, known as the Ida nadi, Pingala nadi and Sushumna nadi. The nadis are located within—but are not of—the physical body. The most important one, the Sushumna runs within the spine. Emerging from the left is the Ida, and from the right is the Pingala. The Ida and pingala are the pathways of the two different aspects of prana. They represent the two opposite poles of the same energy. The ida is denoted as being negative and is also known as the Chandra (~moon) nadi. The Pingala, on the other hand, is positive and often called the Surya (~sun) nadi.

Did you ever ask the question "Why have we got two nostrils?" The Yogi discovered that when the left nostril has the strongest flow of air then the pranic flow in Ida is also predominant. When the right nostril has the greatest flow, Pingala is dominant. The ancient yogi, with their detailed awareness of the human body, found that the flow of breath does not pass equally through each nostril and that the flow of air and prana continually alternates, and influences our lives greatly and consequently so does regulating the flow of breath through these nostrils and the flow of prana through their corresponding pathways. If the right nostril has the greatest flow then we are most likely to be actively inclined and more suited to physical work. When the left nostril has the greater flow, the mind is introverted which is ideal for any kind of mental work.

Rules for pranayama

WE have been breathing all our lives, and there is no harm in pranayama if you use proper breathing techniques without strain. Pranayama can cure disease if done correctly, but if done incorrectly it can cause illness and it is of grave importance that you must develop your abilities slowly and systematically, abiding to the rules here given.

While performing ăsanas correctly, prănăyăma is automatic and without effort along with the movements of the body. The ăsanas herein mentioned have their accompanying breathing technique described for that posture. In prănăyăma, on the other hand, regulation of the mind and body is accomplished through manipulation of the pranic body by means of the breath.

The posture for prănăyăma can be any comfortable sitting position, preferably on a blanket placed on the ground, with the body relaxed and your back kept straight without any strain. Wear light and loose clothing, as circumstances will permit. Let the place of practice be clean, free of strong smells and insects, quiet and properly ventilated so that there is a continuous supply of fresh air. Try to practice in the same place every day, building a quiet and conducive atmosphere. The best time for practice is early morning after ăsanas and before meditation. Be aware of the practice and do not allow it to become automatic. Breathe with control, without any strain and if your mind gets distracted, do not force your mind into obedience. Merely becoming aware of the distraction will direct your attention back to the prănăyăma.

Rhythmic Breathing

THE Yogi knows that by rhythmical breathing one may bring himself into harmonious vibration with nature, and aid in the unfoldment of his latent powers. In rhythmic breathing the main thing to be acquired is the mental idea of rhythm. The Yogi bases his rhythmic breathing time upon a unit corresponding with the beat of his heart. The heart beat varies in different persons, but is the proper rhythmic standard for that particular individual.

Ascertain your normal heart beat by placing your fingers over your pulse, and then count: "1, 2, 3, 4, 5, 6; 1, 2, 3, 4, 5, 6, etc.," until the rhythm becomes firmly fixed in your mind. The beginner usually inhales in about six pulse units, but he will be able to greatly increase this by practice.

The Yogi rule for rhythmic breathing is that the units of inhalation and exhalation should be the same, while the units for retention and between breaths should be one-half the number of those of inhalation and exhalation.

Samaveta Prănăyăma

SAMAVETA' means 'together' and this is a breathing practice where one breathes rhythmically through both nostrils. In other techniques of prănăyăma the flow of air is directed in one nostril by physically or mentally preventing the flow in the other nostril. The following exercise in Samaveta Prănăyăma should be thoroughly mastered before practicing any further forms of prănăyăma, as it forms the basis of many other techniques.

I - Sit upright, in an easy posture, shoulders slightly thrown back and hands resting easily on the lap. In this position, the weight of the body is largely supported by the ribs and may be easily maintained. The Yogi has found that one cannot get the best effect of rhythmic breathing with the chest drawn in and the abdomen protruding.

II - Inhale slowly a Complete Breath, counting six pulse units.

III - Retain, counting three pulse units.

IV - Exhale slowly through the nostrils, counting six pulse units.

V - Count three pulse beats between breaths.

VI - Repeat a number of times, but avoid fatiguing yourself at the start.

After a little practice you will be able to increase the duration of the inhalations and exhalations, until about fifteen pulse units are consumed. In this increase, remember that the units for retention and between breaths are one-half the units for inhalation and exhalation.

Nadi Shodhana Prănăyăma

NADI SHODHANA PRĂNĂYĂMA' purifies the pranic pathways (Nadis) allowing the prana to flow freely throughout your body. Nadi Shodhana is an excellent preparation for more advanced forms of prănăyăma and a very good prelude to meditation or relaxation for it instils calmness of mind. In English this practice can be called the 'Alternate Nostril Prănăyăma,' because the air is inhaled through one nostril and exhaled through the other, nourishing your body with an extra supply of oxygen and more efficiently eliminating the carbon dioxide. This purifies your blood and increases the overall health and resistance to disease.

I - Sit up straight in a comfortable position with the eyes closed, relaxing your whole body. Place your left hand on the left knee in Chin Mudra. Raise your right hand in Nasagra Mudra in front of the face and close the right nostril with the thumb.

II - Inhale through the left nostril (pooraka). Breathe as deeply as possible utilizing the yogi complete breath without straining yourself. At the end of the inhalation, close your left nostril with the ring finger.

III - Now open your right nostril and exhale slowly emptying the lungs completely (rechaka).

IV - At the end of exhalation keep the right nostril open and then slowly inhale. After completing the full yogi breath, close the right nostril.

V - Open the left nostril and exhale.

This is one round. While you do a few rounds like thus, keep your awareness on your breath. After a few breaths, start counting the time of inhalation and exhalation in your mind. Keep the timing of the counting fixed and for the first stage of practice the duration of inhalation equals the time of exhalation. Begin with whatever count you find comfortable whether it is two or ten. Over a period of weeks and months, slowly increase the duration. Practice for as long as time permits, ideally at least ten minutes.

Advancing further into developing your capabilities after mastering the above technique, requires for you to be very disciplined. Make sure not to add a single pulse unit to any given ratio hereafter, before you can practice at your current limit without any sign of strain or effort for the duration of the aforementioned 10 minutes of practice. Be advised and proceed.

VI - The following step in advancing your abilities is to add a holding of the breath (Antar Kumbhaka ~inner breath retention) after each inhalation.

At first, hold the breath for a few pulse units only, and if you feel you have to strain, reduce your count so that the complete round of pranayama becomes comfortable again and can be done without stain. From there continue further, slowly increasing your count and ability to hold your breath over time by adding a pulse unit once you feel utterly comfortable and are performing without strain, until you can hold your breath double the counts as it takes for you to inhale. Ratio 1:2:1 (inhalation: retention: exhalation)

VII - To advance further after mastering the above technique, exhale more slowly until you reach double the amount of counts it takes you to inhale. Ratio 1:2:2.

You aim to master the ratio 1:8:6, which can be achieved by slowly increasing only when you can perform a ratio without strain or effort.

VIII - The next step is to include Bahir kumbhaka (outer retention.) This is something our lungs are not doing quite so often and you should develop this capacity slowly.

At the beginning just add one or two pulse units at the end of an exhalation while you close both nostrils, then to slowly breathe in through the one nostril again. Advance until the ratio will be 1:8:6:1 (inhalation: retention: exhalation: retention)

I - Inhale through left nostril (Pooraka)	—1—
II - Retain breath internally (Antar Kumbhaka)	—8—
III - Exhale through right nostril (Rechaka)	—6—
IV - Retain breath externally (Bahir Kumbhaka)	—1—
V - Inhale through right nostril	—1—
VI - Retain breath internally	—8—
VII - Exhale through left nostril	—6—
VIII - Retain breath externally	—1—

This is one round. Only you will know your capacity, and you must set the number of pulse units of each given ratio to suit your own capabilities.

PART VI

The Science of Relaxation

RELAXATION forms a very important part of the Hatha Yoga philosophy and many of the Yogis have devoted much care and study to this branch of the subject. At first glance, it may appear to the average reader that the idea of teaching people how to relax—how to rest—is ridiculous, as everyone should know how to perform this simple feat. Nature teaches us how to relax and rest to perfection—the infant is a past-master in the science. But as we have grown older we have acquired many artificial habits and have allowed Nature's original habits to lapse.

Our readers are doubtless familiar with the axiom of psychology,

'Thought takes form in action.'

Our first impulse when we wish to do something is to make the muscular movement necessary to the accomplishment of the action proceeding from the thought. But we may be restrained from making the movement by another thought, which shows us the desirability of repressing the action. Inflamed with anger we may experience a desire to strike the person causing the anger, but before the muscle fairly moves our better judgment causes us to send a repressing impulse, and the opposite set of muscles holds back the action of the first set. All this in the fraction of a second. The double action, ordering and countermanding, is performed so quickly that the mind cannot grasp any sense of motion, but nevertheless the muscle had begun to quiver with the striking impulse by the time the restraining impulse operated the opposing set of muscles and held back the movement.

This same principle, carried to still further refinements, causes a slight current of prana to the muscle, and a consequent slight muscular contraction, to follow many unrestrained thoughts, with a constant waste of prana and a perpetual wear and tear upon the nervous system and muscles. Many people of an excitable; irritable, emotional habit of mind constantly keep their nerves in action and their muscles tense by unrestrained and uncontrolled mental states. The person who has naturally, or has cultivated, a calm, controlled mind, will have no such impulses. He moves along well poised and well in hand, and does not allow his thoughts to run away with him. He is a Master, not a slave.

The person understanding Relaxation and the conserving of energy accomplishes the best work. He uses a pound of effort to do the pound of work, and does not waste, or allow his strength to trickle away. The average person not understanding this law uses up from three to twenty-five times the energy needed to do his work, be that work mental or physical. In relaxation the muscles and nerves are at rest, and the prana is being stored up and conserved, instead of being dissipated in reckless expenditures.

Relaxation may be observed in young children, and among the animals. Some adults have it, and such individuals are always noted for their endurance, strength, vigour and vitality.

Rules for Relaxation

THOUGHTS take form in action, and actions react upon the mind. These two truths stand together. One is as true as the other. We have heard much of the influence of the mind over the body, but we must not forget that the body, or its attitudes and positions, react upon the mind and influence mental states. We must remember these two truths in considering the question of relaxation.

One of the first steps toward preventing the harmful practices of muscular contraction, with its resulting waste of prana and wearing out of the nerves is to cultivate a mental attitude of calm and repose. Mental poise and repose may be brought about by the eradication of Worry and Anger. Of course, Fear really underlies both Worry and Anger.

The Yogi considers Anger an unworthy emotion, natural in the lower animals and in savage man but out of place in the developed man. He knows that nothing is accomplished by it, and that it is a useless waste of energy and a positive injury to the brain and nervous system, besides being a weakening element in one's moral nature and spiritual growth. This does not mean that the Yogi is a timid creature without any 'backbone.' On the contrary, he does not know the existence of Fear, and his calmness is instinctively felt to be the indication of strength, not weakness.

The Yogi also has eradicated Worry from his mental condition. He has learned to know that it is a foolish waste of energy, which results in no good and always works harm. He believes in earnest thought when problems have to be solved, obstacles surmounted, but he never descends to Worry. He regards Worry as waste energy and motion, and also as being unworthy of a developed man. He knows his own nature and powers too well to allow himself to worry. He has gradually emancipated himself from its curse and teaches his students that the freeing of oneself from Anger and Worry is the first step in practical Yoga.

While the controlling of the unworthy emotions of the lower nature really form a part of other branches of the Yogi philosophy, it has a direct bearing upon the question of Relaxation, inasmuch as it is a fact that one habitually free from Anger and Worry is correspondingly free from the principal causes of involuntary muscular contraction and nerve-waste. The man possessed by Anger has muscles on the strain from chronic involuntary impulses from the brain. The man who is wrapped in the folds of Worry is constantly in a state of nervous strain and muscular contraction. If you would be free from this great source of waste, manage to get rid of the emotions causing it. And, on the other hand, the practice of relaxing—of avoiding the tense condition of the muscles, in everyday life—will react upon the mind, and will enable it to regain its normal poise and repose. It is a rule that works both ways.

One of the first lessons in physical relaxation the Hatha Yogis give to their pupils is given in the next paragraph. Before beginning, however, we wish to impress upon the mind of the reader the keynote of the Yogi practice of Relaxation. It consists of two words: "LET GO." If you master the meaning of these two words and are able to put them into practice you have grasped the secret of the Yogi Theory and practice of Relaxation.

Relaxation Exercises

THERE are a number of exercises in Relaxation taught and practiced by the Hatha Yogis, the following being among the best. You will start these relaxation exercises from a standing position.

I - Withdraw all prana from the hand, letting the muscles relax so that the hand will swing loosely from the wrist, apparently lifeless. Shake it backward and forwards from the wrist. Then try the other hand the same way. Then both hands together. A little practice will give you the correct idea.

II - Withdraw all prana from the arms and let them hang limp and loose by the sides. Then swing the body from side to side, letting the arms swing (like empty coat-sleeves) from the motion of the body, making no effort of the arms themselves. First one arm and then the other, and then both. This exercise may be varied by twisting the body around in various ways, letting the arms swing loose.

III - Relax the forearm, letting it swing loose from the elbow. Impart a motion from the upper-arm, but avoid contracting the muscles of the forearm. Shake the forearm around limp and loose. First one arm, then the other, then both.

IV - Let the foot be completely relaxed and swung loose from the ankle. This will require some little practice, as the muscles moving the feet are generally in a more or less contracted condition. First one foot, then the other.

V - Relax the leg, withdrawing all prana from it and letting it swing loose and limp from the knee. Then swing it and shake it. First one leg and then the other.

VI - Stand on a cushion, stool or large book and let one leg swing loose and limp from the thigh, after having relaxed it completely. First one leg and then the other.

VII - Raise the arms straight above the head, and then, withdrawing all prana from them, let them drop of their own weight to the sides.

VIII - Lift the knee up in front as high as you can and then draw all prana from it and let it drop back of its own weight.

IX - Relax the head, letting it drop forward, and then swing it about by the motion of the body. Then, sitting back in a chair, relax it and let it drop backward. It will, of course, drop in any direction the moment you withdraw the prana from it. To get the right idea, think of a person falling asleep, who, the moment sleep overpowers him, relaxes and stops contracting the muscles of the neck, allowing the head to drop forward.

X - Relax the muscles of the shoulders and chest, allowing the upper part of the chest to fall forward loose and limp.

XI - Sit in a chair and relax the muscles of the waist, which will allow the upper part of the body to pitch forward like that of a child who falls asleep in its chair and gradually falls out.

One who has mastered these exercises so far may, if he sees fit, relax his whole body, commencing with the neck, until he gets down to the knees, when he will drop gently to the floor 'all in a heap.' This is a valuable acquirement, as in case of one slipping or falling by accident. The practice of this entire body relaxation will do much to protect from injury. You will notice that a young child will relax in this way when it falls, and is scarcely affected by severe falls which would seriously bruise adults, or even break their limbs. The same phenomenon may be noticed in the cases of intoxicated persons who have lost control of the muscles and are in an almost complete state of relaxation. When they fall they come down 'all in a heap' and suffer comparatively little injury.

In practicing these exercises repeat each of them several times and then pass on to the next one. These exercises may be almost indefinitely extended and varied, according to the ingenuity and power of invention of the student. Make your own exercises, if you will, using the above as suggestions.

Practicing relaxation exercises, gives one a consciousness of self-control and repose, which is valuable. Strength in repose is the idea to be carried in the mind when thinking of the Yogi Relaxation theories. It is useful in quieting overwrought nerves; is an antidote for what is known as 'muscle-bound' conditions resulting from the employment of certain sets of muscles in one's daily work or exercise, and is a valuable acquirement in the direction of allowing one to rest himself at will and to thus regain his vitality in the shortest possible time.

Nearly all the wandering races and tribes have acquired this knowledge. They will undertake journeys which would frighten a civilized man, and after travelling many miles will make a resting place, upon which they will throw themselves down, relaxing every muscle and withdrawing the prana from all the voluntary muscles, allowing themselves to remain limp and apparently lifeless from head to foot. They indulge in a doze at the same time, if practicable, but if not they remain wide awake, with senses active and alert, but with the bodily muscles as above stated. One hour of this rest refreshes them as much, or more, than a night's sleep does the average man. They start on their journey again, refreshed and with new life and energy.

It seems to have been intuitively acquired by the American Indian, the Arab, the savage tribes of Africa, and, in fact, races in all parts of the world. Civilized man has allowed this gift to lapse, because he has ceased to make the long journeys on foot, but it would be well for him to regain this lost knowledge and use it to relieve the fatigue and nerve-exhaustion of the strenuous business life, which has taken the place of the old wandering life, with all its hardships.

Relaxation Through Stretching

STRETCHING is another method of resting employed by the Yogis. At first sight this will seem to be the reverse of relaxation, but it is really akin to it, as it withdraws the tension from the muscles which have been habitually contracted. Nature impels us to yawn and stretch when we are fatigued. Let us take a lesson from her book. Let us learn to stretch at will as well as involuntarily. This is not as easy as you may imagine and you will have to practice somewhat before you get the full benefit from it.

Take up the Relaxation exercises in the order in which they are given in this chapter, but instead of relaxing each part in turn simply stretch them. Begin with the feet, and then work up to the legs, and then up to the arms and head. Stretch in all sorts of ways, twisting your legs, feet, arms, hands, head and body around in a way you feel like to get the full benefit of the stretch. Don't be afraid of yawning, either; that is simply one form of stretch. In stretching you will, of course, tense and contract muscles, but the rest and relief comes in the subsequent relaxation of them. Carry in your mind the 'let-go' idea, rather than that of muscular exertion. We cannot attempt to give exercises in stretching, as the variety open to the student is so great that he should not require to have illustrations given him. Just let him give way to the mental idea of a good, restful stretch, and Nature will tell him what to do. Here is one general suggestion, however:

1. Stand on the floor, with your legs spread apart and your arms extended over your head, also spread apart. Then raise yourself on your toes and stretch yourself out gradually as if you were trying to reach the ceiling. A most simple exercise, but wonderfully refreshing.

All of these plans of relaxing, if properly entered into and carried out will leave the one practicing them with a sense of renewed energy and an inclination to again resume work, the same feeling as one experiences after arising from a healthy sleep and a subsequent good rubdown in the bath.

Mental Relaxation

OF course, physical relaxation reacts on the mind and rests it. But mental relaxation also reacts upon the body and rests it. So this exercise may reach the needs of some who have not found just what they required in the preceding pages of this section.

Sit quietly in a relaxed and easy position and withdraw the mind as far as possible from outside objects or thoughts which require active mental effort. Let your thought reach inward and dwell upon the real self. Think of yourself as independent of the body and as able to leave it without impairing the individuality. You will gradually experience a feeling of blissful rest and calm and content. The attention must be withdrawn entirely from the physical body and centered entirely upon the higher 'I,' which is really 'you.' Think of the vast worlds around us, the millions of suns, each surrounded with its group of planets like our earth, only in many cases much larger. 'Get an idea of the immensity of space and of time; consider the extent of Life in all its forms in all these worlds and then realize the position of the earth and of yourself a mere insect upon a speck of dirt. Then rise upward in your thought and realize that, though you be but an atom of the mighty whole, you are still a bit of Life itself, a particle of the Spirit; that you are immortal, eternal and indestructible; a necessary part of the Whole, a part which the Whole cannot get along without, a piece needed to fit into the structure of the Whole. Recognize yourself as in touch with all of Life; feel the Life of the Whole throbbing through you; the whole ocean of Life rocking you on its bosom. And then awake and return to your physical life and you will find that your body is refreshed, your mind calm and strong, and you will feel an inclination to do that piece of work which you have been putting off for so long. You have profited and been strengthened by your trip into the upper regions of the mind.

Savǎsana

CORPSE POSE.' Following asana is a favorite Yogi exercise in relaxation. Performed to its perfection the Savǎsana incorporates all the elements of the rules for relaxation and relaxation exercises mentioned earlier. Savǎsana can be practiced anytime, and should surely be practiced after yoga exercises and ǎsanas.

Savǎsana removes physical as well as mental fatigue, and has been accorded a pride of place in the science of yoga. Savǎsana is a unique feature of the yogic system of exercises and is unparalleled by any other exercise, being a process in which not only is there no active contractile tension generated in the motor organs of the body, but an attempt at active relaxation is made to include every part of the body.

It has to be performed by all yogis, amateurs and adepts alike, because, without this asana, the fatigue generated in the minute nerves and tissues by the performance of various yoga exercises and pranayama cannot be relieved; it is the Savǎsana alone which can remove it. The yogis also utilize this asana for the attainment of Samadhi (a state of deep meditation).

Don't lie on a soft bed or mattress as this will not allow you to distinguish whether you are relaxing the muscles or not. If the atmosphere is cold or if there are any small insects in the air, cover yourself with a lightweight, large sheet or blanket. If you feel tension in your back when you lie down, you can bend your knees and pull them tight to your chest before placing them back to the floor. You will feel that your back muscles are now more relaxed and at ease. If you are suffering from back pain or back injuries, bend your knees and place your feet a foot away from your hips. This will support and relax your back.

Try not to move your body at all during the practice, for even the slightest movement will tense muscles. The whole body has to be relaxed and it has to be ensured that not even the smallest part of the body remains tense, to the extent of a feeling of being separated from the body.

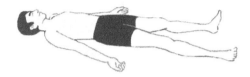

I - Lie flat on your back. Relax as thoroughly as you can, letting go of all the muscles. If you wish, you can place a small pillow behind your head to ensure that your neck and shoulder muscles can relax. Rest the arms on each side of the body leaving a little space between the arms and the side of the body with your palms facing upwards and the hands relaxed. Your legs are straight and slightly separated with the feet fallen to the outside. Close your eyes.

II - While lying relaxed carry in your mind that you are lying on a soft, downy couch and that your body and limbs are as heavy as lead. Repeat the words several times, slowly: *"Heavy as lead, heavy as lead,"* at the same time lifting and tensing the arms making a fist, and then withdrawing the prana from them by ceasing to contract the muscles, and allowing them to drop of their own weight to the sides. After the arms try the legs, one at a time lifting and tensing them. Let them drop of their own weight and remain perfectly relaxed. Then lift the buttocks followed by your chest, allowing them to drop in the same way. Your head is next and tense your facial muscles, open your mouth and stretch your tongue while you exhale forcefully through the mouth. Relax your head on the ground, relax your facial muscles and slowly move your head from left to right, right to left. If you do this thoroughly (you will improve by practice) you will end by having every muscle in the body fully relaxed and the nerves at rest.

III - Then lie still and form the mental image of the couch, or floor, bearing the entire weight of the body. You may laugh at this idea, believing that when you lie down you always let the floor bear all of your weight, but you are mistaken. You will find that, in spite of yourself, you are endeavouring to support a part of your weight by tensing some of the muscles—you are trying to hold yourself up. Take a few deep abdominal breaths, lying quietly and fully relaxed.

IV - Feel the different parts of your body in contact with the floor. Feel that your whole body is very heavy and that it is sinking into the floor. Move your attention to the tips of your toes and mentally feel them become limp and relaxed, and then forget about them completely. This mental relaxation of that body part is followed by moving your attention to your ankles, your calves and your thighs. Proceed to your hips, lower back, and your upper back, all the way forgetting about that part you just so mentally relaxed. Then, address all your internal organs individually. Your small intestine; your large intestine, your pancreas, liver, stomach, kidneys, your heart and your lungs. All your organs are now fully relaxed. Feel the relaxation. Then relax your abdomen, your chest and your arms. Mentally relax your hands, the palms of your hands, relax your fingers. Your shoulders, neck and your chin are completely relaxed. Relax your facial muscles, your eyes, ears and mouth. Your whole head is relaxed now.

V - Feel the relaxation in your whole body. You have no worries or tension. You are completely relaxed.

VI - Become aware of the air touching the tip of your nose. While you breathe in, cool air is touching your nostrils and when you breathe out, warm air is coming out from your nostrils. Remain thus relaxed and aware of the breath for several minutes.

VII - When you finish the practice, gently come to body consciousness; move and clench your hands, move your arms. Move your feet and legs. Slowly open your eyes, turn to the side and sit up. Sit in any comfortable position and relax.

Meditation

THIS work is not intended to delve deep into the higher philosophies of Yoga. However, one of the main goals of the instructions in Hatha Yoga is for the physical body to become an optimal functioning organism that will not interfere with Meditational practices, but rather be supportive of it. For that purpose it will be good to briefly touch upon the subject of Meditation, for its meaning is widely misunderstood.

Each of us has reached a certain point in our evolution, yet at the same time our present condition and values seem to be insufficient. Something is missing from our lives. This missing link is inner, spiritual growth. Evolution is a continuous progression from the unrefined to the refined, from the disorderly to the orderly and from the gross to the subtle. Though separated in time and place, different languages and social backgrounds, the saints, prophets, mystics, sages and yogis who have existed in all places, eras and in all societies all knew that the path each of us must tread lies in awakening our inner potential.

Christ said,

"The kingdom of God is within you."

Buddha said,

"Look within, thou art the Buddha."

The Greeks wrote above the main door of their temples,

"Man, know thyself, and thou shalt know the universe."

In the Bhagavad Gita, Lord Krishna affirmed:

"Meditation is far better than (intellectual) knowledge."

There are many more examples like these. They were speaking about the same basic truth of existence. These people knew that the path of evolution to higher awareness lies in unfolding the inner realms of our being and that infinite dormant potential exists within each of us. To find it, however, we must plunge into our inner being.

The aim of Yoga is to bring the unconscious and subconscious to conscious perception—in Union (Yoga). Only by knowing the depths of the mind can we really know ourselves. The journey into these layers of consciousness requires a vehicle—the vehicle is Meditation. The aim of meditation practices is to induce this 'State of Meditation.'

It is impossible to teach or define the state of Meditation. What can be taught is a method that will lead you to it. The experience of Meditation is not only confined to those who sit in a quiet place with their eyes closed to introspect and induce meditation, the method called 'Raja Yoga.' It is also possible while performing everyday duties. This is more in line with the practices of 'Karma Yoga' and 'Bhakti Yoga.' A person can perform the most trivial actions and yet simultaneously be in the highest state of meditation.

Meditation Techniques

OUR attention on meditation for the sake of this work on Hatha Yoga will be related to 'Raja Yoga.' These techniques are reasonably easy to learn but will never bring results unless they are practised regularly with aspiration and dedication. A fixed period of time is set aside daily solely for the purpose of introspection. There is no need to fill the mind with a variety of different techniques. By practicing one seriously, all is gained and you will experience the joy and knowledge of Meditation.

Many people sit down, close their eyes for some time and consider that they have meditated. Generally one broods over problems and thinks of external happenings while in this so-called state of meditation. Though the eyes may be closed, there is no introspection if the mind is thinking about the outside world. Meditation is beyond this inner—or outer interaction with the world.

The first step is to overcome disturbances of the body. It is difficult for most people to sit comfortably in one position for more than a minute or so without feeling pain or wanting to scratch. Follow the precepts set forth in this book faithfully and all your discomforts will soon be a thing of the past.

The next step is to achieve calmness of mind and relaxation. This is done through awareness. We try to be aware of one object, symbol or process of thought. There are many things that can be used as an object to meditate upon. It does not matter as long as the object is able to hold one's attention easily. A few of the most common are; the breathing process, mantras (such as 'Aum'), an external or internal picture of a God, a sage, a guru, the tip of the nose, different parts of the body or any other symbol that appeals to you. One particularly good practice utilizes awareness of the thought process itself. The vehicle in Karma Yoga is intense, concentrated work; in Bhakti Yoga overwhelming devotion to a person or one object and in Gnani Yoga the vehicle is an all absorbing enquiry. Remember, all these are the means that lead to meditation, not meditation itself.

This takes practice, but eventually it is possible to focus the awareness on one thing to the exclusion of all others. One-pointed attention allows the awareness to pierce and enter the depths of the mind. Furthermore, this one-pointed awareness prevents falling into a state of unconsciousness, sleep when one meditates. Concentration does not come easily or spontaneously. Be aware of an object or process of thought to the best of your ability, don't fight the wandering mind—let it wander, but remain aware of what you have chosen as your object of meditation. In this way you will not only attain one-pointedness but will simultaneously enjoy a state of mental and physical relaxation.

Meditational practices are excellent methods of confronting the problems, conflicts and other disturbances hidden in the recesses of the mind. Once we face these negative aspects of our mind they will automatically drop away. As these problems are gradually removed, so one's life becomes an expression of joy and happiness. Our lives will be transformed. It is possible for everyone to know the joy of meditation, yet at the same time effort is required. It would be most surprising if a person starts to meditate on the first attempt. Regular and sincere practice and time are required. All effort is worthwhile, no matter how long or short the practice may be. More so than anything else you are likely to do in your life.

Don't expect instant meditation but persevere in your practices. It is only personal experience of meditation, even if it is the faintest glimmer, that can make us realize the power, knowledge and joy that is our heritage. We encourage our readers to seek more knowledge about the subjects touched upon in this chapter by exploring the higher teachings to be found in the wisdom of the Threefold Path. For the purpose of this work the here mentioned guidelines will suffice, and we will close the subject by giving you some ways of sitting best suited for meditational practices.

Siddhăsana

MALE ACCOMPLISHED POSE.' Siddhăsana can be practised by men. The female equivalent is called Siddha Yoni Ăsana. This Asana is often used in specific practices for it applies pressure in the region between the anus and the sexual organs. This pressure is important, for it is concerned with awakening a psychic centre in this area (mooladhara chakra). The practice of this asana helps to check sensuality and attain Brahmacarya. (The word 'Brahmacarya,' though meaning a vow of celibacy in common use, indicates also the state of the mind concentrated on the Supreme Being). This asana provides mental discipline and ensures the passage of the Prana in the Sushumna Nadi. It thus helps in the awakening of Kundalini Sakti (Serpent power). It is possible to attain Dharana (concentration) Dhyana (meditation) and even Samadhi (contemplation and self realisation) through this asana. Different results are obtained by fixing the gaze in different ways:

I - Bhru-madhya-drsti (gazing at the centre of the eyebrows), produces a vision of lights.

II - Sama-drsti (looking straight ahead) is especially useful for those practising Trataka or central fixation.

III - Nasikagra-drsti (gazing at the tip of the nose) gives a vision of the 5 elements of which the Universe is composed (in Samkhya-Yoga.)

These are the Akasa, Vayu, Tejas, Ap and Prithvi. Although, usually and loosely translated as ether, air, light, water and earth, these synonyms fail to convey the philosophical and metaphysical import of the original terms, which, rather than denoting any particular substance, merely connote different basic types and stages of organisation of matter. For a proper appreciation of these terms a standard text on Indian philosophy should be consulted.

IV- Ardhonmesa (half-open eye lids) helps in promoting the Sambhavi and Unmani poses or Mudras, which should be learnt through a teacher.

V- Netrabandha (closed eyes) is especially helpful for meditation and is, therefore, essential for those whose minds are unsteady and undisciplined.

Those who can maintain the pose continuously for a period of three hours and forty-eight minutes can be considered to have mastered it. This asana should be practiced in moderation by the family man; only yogis should practice it beyond that limit. There are two ways in which the hands can be engaged while performing Siddhăsana.

I- The hands are kept in the lap. This leads to the enhancement of Laghima-Sakti, that is- the body gets lighter.

II- If the hands are kept on the knees, palms upturned and the forefinger bent against the thumb, Garima-Sakti is enhanced and the body gets heavier.

In the beginning, the yogi should strive for the enhancement of Laghima-Sakti and the hands should be kept in the lap. But a time comes when the yogi finds himself being buoyed up, and, if he wants to suppress this buoyancy, he must increase the Garima-Sakti.

Siddhăsana is an excellent meditative ăsana and the equal of Padmăsana.

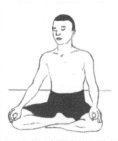

I - Sit on the floor with the sole of your right foot against the inside of the left thigh, and press your right heel against the perineum (area between the anus and the genitals).

II - Place the left foot on top of the right calf and press the left heel into the pelvis so that your genitals lie between the two heels.

III - Push the left toes into the space between your right calf and thigh and grasp your right toes, either from below or above your left leg and pull them upwards into the space between your left thigh and calf.

IV - Adjust the body so that it is comfortable. Take care that the knees are touching the floor and the heels are one above the other. Hold your spine and head upright. Alternate the position of the right- and left leg with each practice.

Siddha Yoni Āsana

ACCOMPLISHED POSE FOR WOMEN.' Yoni ~womb. This āsana is the female equivalent of Siddhāsana and is to be practiced by women. In the instructions for Siddhāsana, adjust your right heel so that it presses firmly against the front of your vagina (labia majora). Adjust your body position so that you are comfortable, while simultaneously feeling the pressure of the right heel.

Padmāsana

LOTUS POSE.' Although difficult, most who practice 'Padmāsana are capable of perfecting it. The Lotus Pose is used for meditation, prayer, worship and pranayama. This asana relieves constipation, indigestion and flatulence. It improves digestion and strengthens the thighs and calves. It is considered more useful to women than to men because it has a beneficial effect on the womb. Therefore, all the āsanas based on Padmăsana should be specially practiced by women.

The pose holds the trunk of the body and the head as though they are a pillar, with the legs as its firm foundation. The position and pressure of the feet against the thighs reduces the flow of blood to the legs which is redirected towards the abdominal and pelvic organs and nerves in the region. The yogi seats himself in Padmăsana and practices pranayama. We mention pranayama here because perfect pranayama can be performed only in Padmăsana. This is also one of the best meditative āsanas, and with practice will prove far more comfortable than simpler sitting positions with the added distinction in that it is decidedly more effective and useful than siddhăsana for physical well-being.

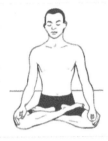

I - Sit on the floor with your left leg on the right thigh with the sole of your foot facing up with the heel touching the front of the lower abdomen as close as possible to the navel.

II - Fold the other leg in the same way and place the foot on top of the opposite thigh in such a way that the heels touch each other as near the navel as possible. Both knees rest comfortably on the floor. Relax your arms with the elbows bent, keep your back and head upright and your hands on the knees or in the lap with the palms facing up. Close your eyes and relax. This is the final pose.

III - The whole procedure is to be repeated by altering the sequence in which the feet are placed on the thighs.

IV - You can practice a number of mudras. Two important ones are jnana mudra and chin mudra.

Keeping the hands in the lap causes the body to get lighter (Laghima-Sakti). Keeping the hands on the knees enhances the effect of gravity, and the body gets heavier. In the beginning the yogi should try to cultivate the Laghima-Sakti and the hands should be kept in the lap.

A more easy variation and an excellent ǎsana to prepare the legs for Padmǎsana, is the half lotus pose, Ardha Padmǎsana. It is also a very good meditative ǎsana in its own right. It is a good pose for your hips, knees and ankles, giving you more flexibility and with regular practice you can accomplish the Padmǎsana.

I - Sit on the floor with the legs extended in front of the body.

II - Bend your right knee and place the right foot on top of your left thigh with the sole facing upwards.

III - Then bend your left knee and place your left foot under your right thigh. You are now sitting in a half lotus pose.

IV - Adjust your body to a comfortable position. Hold your back, neck and head upright. Place the hands on the knees or in the lap, close your eyes and relax.

V - You can sit for some minutes in this pose and then change your legs, or change when the position becomes uncomfortable. If you prefer to remain seated, then next time you sit for practice, place the other leg on top.

Once you have mastered Padmǎsana, there is a variety of ǎsanas you can perform with each their own specific benefits and effect on the body.

Veerǎsana

HERO'S POSE' The large area of contact with the ground makes the Veerǎsana a comfortable sitting position for those people who cannot sit in the more difficult meditative ǎsanas. You can alternate which leg is positioned at the bottom and which one on top.

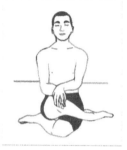

I - Sit with your legs outstretched in front of the body.

II - Bend your left leg and place the left foot under and to the side of the right buttock.

III - Bend your right leg over the top of the left leg, placing the right foot beside the left buttock. Arrange the position of the knees so that one is above the other.

IV - Hold the head, neck and back upright. Place the hands in a most comfortable position in which your arms are relaxed.

Vajrăsana

ANKLE POSE.' From Sanskrit Vajra translates into "thunderbolt" or "diamond like". Figuratively Vajra signifies strength and vigour. The body gets strong and firm from the practice of this asana. Hence the yogis have named it Vajrăsana, implying that through its practice the body becomes like a diamond. It loosens the joints and muscles of the legs, the knees, the ankles and the toes, making them strong and flexible and preventing flat foot. The Vajra nadi which runs through the ankle is positively affected, and blood circulation to the lower abdominal region increases. Practice Vajrăsana after meals, when the flow of the nadis is usually downwards. The asana reverses this flow and thus helps in the speedy digestion of food. It is the only posture which can be performed even after heavy food. It is a very useful asana for meditation and pranayama practices. It keeps the spine erect and prevents drowsiness.

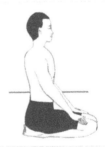

I - Sit straight with your legs stretched and the heels together, with the palms of your hands pressing on the floor by the side of the buttocks.

II - Fold the right leg at the knee and place the heel under the right buttock. Then do the same with the left leg.

III - Keep your knees and heels together, and rest the palms of your hands on the upper thighs. Sit with your spine straight, your shoulders and neck relaxed. This is the final pose. To come out from it, reverse the steps.

PART VIII

Săntih Mantras

PEACE MANTRAS' are prayers for Peace. Săntih Mantras are to calm the mind and the environment. Reciting them is also believed to be removing any obstacles for the task ahead. Săntih Mantras always end with three utterances of the word 'Săntih' which means 'Peace.' The reason for uttering this word three times is for calming and removing obstacles in the three realms called 'Tapa-Traya' or three classes of obstacles, which are:

I - The 'Physical' world or 'Adhi-Bhautika.' This is the source of obstacles coming from the external world, such as wild animals, people, natural calamities etc.

II - The 'Divine' world or 'Adhi-Daivika.' Obstacles that come from the extra-sensory world of spirits, ghosts, deities, demigods etc.

III - The 'Internal' world or 'Adhyaatmika,' obstacles arising out of one's own body and mind, such as pain, diseases, laziness, absent-mindedness etc.

Sāntih Mantra I

Om Saha Năvavatu,
Om! May He protect us both together;

Saha Nau Bhunaktu,
May He nourish us both together;

Saha Vīryam Karavăvahai,
May we work conjointly with great energy,

Tejasvi năvadhĭtamastu,
May our study be vigorous and effective;

Mă Vidviṣăvahai,
May we not hate any.

Om Śăntih Śăntih Śăntih
Om! Peace Peace Peace

Sāntih Mantra II

Om Pŭrnamadah,
Om! That is infinite (Brahman),

Pŭrnamidam,
and this (universe) is infinite.

Pŭrnăt Pŭrnamudacyate,
The infinite proceeds from the infinite.

Pŭrnasya Pŭrnamădăya,
(Then) taking the infinitude of the infinite (universe).

Pŭrnamevăvaśisyate,
It remains as the infinite (Brahman) alone.

Om Śăntih Śăntih Śăntih
Om! Peace Peace Peace

Lead by the Spirit

WHILE this book is intended to treat solely upon the care of the physical body, leaving the higher branches of the Yogi Philosophy to be dealt with in other writings, still the leading principle of the Yogi teachings is so bound up with the minor branches of the subject, and is so largely taken into account by the Yogis in the simplest acts of their lives, that in justice to the teachings, we cannot leave the subject without at least saying a few words about this underlying principle.

The Yogi Philosophy holds that man is slowly growing and unfolding, from the lower forms and manifestations to higher, and still higher expressions of the Spirit. Spirit is in each man, although often so obscured by the confining sheaths of his lower nature that it is scarcely discernible. It is also in the lower forms of life, working up and ever seeking for higher forms of expression. The material sheaths of this progressing life—bodies of mineral, plant, lower animal and man—are but instruments to be used for the best development of the higher principles. Although the use of the material body is only temporary and the body itself nothing more than a suit of clothes to be put on, worn, and then discarded, yet it is always the intent of Spirit to provide and maintain as perfect an instrument as possible. It provides the best body possible, and gives the impulses toward right living, but if from causes not to be mentioned here, an imperfect body is provided for the soul, still the higher principles strive to adapt and accommodate themselves to it, and make the best of it.

This instinct of self-preservation—this urge behind all of life—is a manifestation of the Spirit. It works through the most rudimentary forms of the Instinctive Mind up through many stages until it reaches the highest manifestations of that mental principle. It also manifests through the Intellect, in the direction of causing the man to use his reasoning powers for the purpose of maintaining his physical soundness and life. But, alas! The Intellect does not keep to its own work, for as soon as it begins to be conscious of itself it begins to meddle with the duties of the Instinctive Mind, and overriding the instinct of the latter, it forces all sort of unnatural modes of living upon the body. It is like a boy freed from the parental restraint, which goes as far contrary to the parents' example and advice as possible—just to show that he is independent. But the boy learns his folly, and retraces his steps—and so will the Intellect.

Man is now beginning to see that there is something within him that attends to the wants of his body, and which knows its own business much better than he does. For Man with all his Intellect is unable to duplicate the feats of the Instinctive Mind working through the body of the plant, animal or himself. And he learns to trust this mental principle as a friend, and to let it work out its own duties. In the present modes of life which Man has adopted in his evolution, t is impossible to live a wholly natural life, and physical existence must be more or less abnormal as a consequence. However, Nature's instinct of self-preservation and accommodation is great, and it manages to get along very well with a considerable handicap, and does its work much better than one would expect considering the absurd and insane living habits and practices of civilized Man.

From this, Man will return to first principles sooner or later. It must not be forgotten, that as Man advances along the scale and the Spiritual Mind begins to unfold, Man acquires something akin to Instinct—we call it Intuition—and this leads him back to nature. We can see the influence of this dawning consciousness in the movement back toward natural living and the simple life, which is growing so rapidly the last few years. We are beginning to laugh at the absurd forms, conventions and fashions which have grown up around our civilization and which, unless we get rid of them, will pull down that civilization beneath its growing weight.

The man and woman in whom the Spiritual Mind is unfolding, will become dissatisfied with the artificial life and customs, and will find a strong inclination to return to simpler and more natural principles of living, thinking and acting, and will grow impatient under the restraint and artificial coverings and bandages with which man has bound himself during the ages. He will feel the homing instinct—'after long ages we are coming home." And the Intellect will respond, and seeing the follies it has perpetrated, will endeavour to 'let go' and return to nature, doing its own work all the better by reason of having allowed the Instinctive Mind to attend to its own work without meddling.

The whole theory and practice of Hatha Yogi is based upon this idea of return to nature—the belief that the Instinctive Mind of man contains that which will maintain health under normal conditions. And accordingly those who practice its teachings learn first to 'let go,' and then to live as closely to natural conditions as is possible in this age of artificiality.

We are not unmindful of the fact that it is much harder for the man and woman to adopt natural methods of living, when all their surroundings impel them the other way, but still each may do a little each day for himself and the race, in this direction, and it is surprising how the old artificial habits will drop from a person—one by one.

In this our concluding chapter, we wish to impress upon you the fact that one may be led by the Spirit in the physical life, as well as in the mental. One may implicitly trust the Spirit to guide him in the right way in the matter of everyday living as well as in the more complicated matters of life. If one will trust in the Spirit, he will find that his old appetites will drop away from him—his abnormal tastes will disappear— and he will find a joy and pleasure in the simpler living which will make life seem like a different thing to him.

One should not attempt to separate his belief in the Spirit from his physical life—for Spirit pervades everything, and manifests in the physical (or rather through it) as well as in the highest mental states. One may eat with the Spirit and drink with it, as well as think with it. It will not do to say *this is spiritual, and that is not,* for all is spiritual, in the highest sense.

If one wishes to make the most of his physical life—to have as perfect an instrument as may be for the expression of the Spirit—let him live his life all the way through in that trust and confidence in the spiritual part of his nature. Let him realize that the Spirit within him is a spark from the Divine Flame—a drop from the Ocean of Spirit—a ray from the Central Sun. Let him realize that he is an eternal being—always growing, developing and unfolding. Always moving toward the great goal the exact nature of which man, in his present state, is unable to grasp with his imperfect mental vision. The urge is always onward and upward. We are all a part of that great Life which is manifesting itself in infinitude of infinitude of forms and shapes. We are all a part of IT. If we can but grasp the faintest idea of what this means, we will open ourselves up to such an influx of Life and vitality that our bodies will be practically made over and will manifest perfectly. Let each of us form an idea of a Perfect Body, and endeavour to so live that we will grow into its physical form—and we can do this.

We have tried to tell you the laws governing the physical body, that you may conform to them as near as may be—interposing as little friction as possible to the inflow of that great Life and Energy which is anxious to flow through us. Let us return to nature, and allow this great life to flow through us freely, and all will be well with us. Let us stop trying to do the whole thing ourselves—let us just LET the thing do its own work for us. It only asks confidence and non-resistance

—let us give it a chance.

Om
Śăntih
Śăntih
Śăntih

∽◎ PART X ◎∽

Appendix

Daily Practice Program

Sit comfortably in a meditation pose

Săntih Mantra I .... Prayer for Peace I

Breathing Exercises

Hand in- and out breathing..Breathing exercise
Hand stretch breathing ....Breathing exercise
Ankles stretch breathing ....Breathing exercise

Ăsanas

Sŭrya Namaskăra [6 rounds]...Sun Salutation
Trikonăsana *or* Părsvakonăsana...............................Triangle- *or* Side Angle Pose
Pada Hastasana ....Forward Bending Pose
Ardha Chakrăsana ....Half Wheel Pose
Vrkshasana- Garudăsana *or* Natarăjăsana .... Tree-, Eagle- *or* Lord Dance Pose
Sirsăsana (For advanced practitioners) ....Headstand Pose
Utthanpadăsana [5 times each] ....Raised Leg Pose
Cross-legged Lumbar stretch..Stretching exercise
Sarvăngăsana...Shoulder Stand
Halăsana ....Plough Pose
Matsyăsana...Fish Pose
Purvottanăsana ....Inclined Plane Pose
Chakrăsana ....Wheel Pose
Pavana muktăsana ....Wind Release Pose
Pascimottănăsana.. Back Stretching Pose
Purvottanăsana *or* Ustrăsana........................... Inclined Plane- *or* Camel Pose
Gomukhăsana ....Cow's Face Pose
Makarăsana..Crocodile Pose
Bhujangăsana [2 times] ....Cobra Pose
Ardha Shalabhăsana [2 times] ....Half Locust Pose
Shalabhăsana [2 times] .... Locust Pose
Dhanurăsana [2 times] ....Bow Pose
Balăsana...Child Pose
Meru Vakrăsana *or* Ardha Matsyendrăsana...................... Spinal- *or* Half Spinal Twist
Kakăsana..Crow Pose
Mayurăsana (For advanced practitioners) ....Peacock Pose
Titli Ăsana ....Butterfly Pose

Prănăyăma, relaxation and meditation

Kapălabhăti..Frontal Brain Cleansing
Nadi Shodhana Prănăyăma ....Alternate Nostril Prănăyăma
Savăsana..Corpse Pose
Săntih Mantra II.. Prayer for Peace II
Meditate in a comfortable pose for as long as time permits............................

Index of subjects

Index of exercises